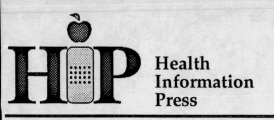

Health Information Press

Corporate Office
4727 Wilshire Boulevard
Los Angeles, CA 90010

Phone: 213-954-0224
Fax: 213-954-0253

Review Slip

The Patient's Guide to Medical Terminology
Translating the Confusing Language of Medicine into Easy-to-Understand English, Third Edition

by Charlotte Isler

208 pages 6" x 9"

$12.95 trade paperback

ISBN: 1-885987-08-0

Category: Health / Medical Reference

Publication date: August 1997

Please send two copies of any review or mention to
Health Information Press
4727 Wilshire Blvd, Los Angeles, CA 90010

For additional information, please contact:
Kate Bandos, KSB Promotions
1-800-304-3269 or 616-676-0758
fax 616-676-0759 • e-mail: KSBPromo@aol.com

The Patient's Guide to Medical Terminology is available at bookstores or directly from Health Information Press by calling 1-800-MED-SHOP.

THIRD EDITION

THE PATIENT'S GUIDE TO MEDICAL TERMINOLOGY

CHARLOTTE ISLER

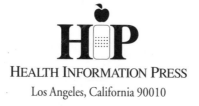

HEALTH INFORMATION PRESS

Los Angeles, California 90010

Library of Congress Cataloging-in-Publication Data

Isler, Charlotte
    [The Patient's guide to medical terminology]
    Isler's patient guide to medical terminology /
    Charlotte Isler. -- Rev. 3rd ed.
         p. cm. -- (PMIC Consumer health series)
    Previously published as: Isler's pocket dictionary.
    ISBN 1-57066-004-2
    1. Medicine--Dictionaries. 2. Medicine, Popular--Dictionaries.
    I. Isler, Charlotte. Isler's pocket dictionary. II. Title.
    III. Series.
    R121.I85 1994
    610'.3--dc20   94-39738   CIP

ISBN 1-885987-08-0

Health Information Press
4727 Wilshire Blvd., Suite 300
Los Angeles, CA 90010

Printed in the United States of America

CONTENTS

Preface v

How to Use this Book 1

Section 1: Abbreviations 5

Section 2: Definitions 39
    A 39
    B 61
    C 69
    D 93
    E 101
    F 113
    G 121
    H 131
    I 145
    J 155
    K 157
    L 161
    M 169
    N 177
    O 181
    P 185
    Q 203
    R 205
    S 213
    T 225
    U 239
    V 243
    W 251
    XYZ 253

Measures and Equivalents 255

About the Author 257

PREFACE

Have you ever left a doctor's office after being told you need a certain test, only to discover by the time you got home that you can't remember its exact name or even its purpose? Many patients have that experience; most are too embarrassed to call the doctor back and admit that they've forgotten what they've just been told.

There is no mystery as to why this happens: For one thing, you and other patients are understandably nervous when you visit the doctor, concerned about a particular health complaint. For another, you've probably never heard any of the medical terms and abbreviations commonly used by health professionals as they discuss tests, diagnostic procedures and different diseases. It's "medicalese" only they can understand, and they often forget that their language is "Greek" to you.

Instead of feeling better when you leave your doctor's office, you may end up feeling worse; you still don't know what's wrong with you, and you've forgotten which tests the doctor wants you to have, and why. Yet obviously, you have every right to know what's going on inside your body, and the doctor's plans for your healthcare. That's where this **Patient Guide** will help.

This book provides brief, clear descriptions of common illnesses, diagnostic tests, terms, and procedures. If you remember only a word or an abbreviation following a doctor's visit, just consult the appropriate section of this guide, as explained in **"How To Use This Book"** (page ix), for an exact, easy to understand description.

Then, when you or a family member need to see the doctor again, ask further questions about your tests and treatment, and (pencil and pad at the ready to write down the answers), find out exactly where you stand. If further tests or other procedures are needed, consult this guide again to stay fully informed and find out how the doctor intends to solve the problem.

— Charlotte Isler

HOW TO USE THIS BOOK

There are three sections contained in this consumer guide:
    Section 1: Abbreviations
    Section 2: Definitions
    Section 3: Measures and Equivalents.

If you already know the name of the term, disease, diagnostic test or procedure, simply look it up in *Section 2: Definitions*. Here you will find all entries listed in alphabetical order.

If you have only a word or abbreviation for a test, term or procedure, but you don't know the meaning, start with *Section 1: Abbreviations*. This will provide you with the complete word(s) or term(s). Then you can proceed to Section 2, which will explain the word or term.

The normal values for any given test may vary for several reasons. First, there is a normal range of values, since no two individuals react alike to any given test. Second, test results vary depending on the laboratory method used, and on the laboratory itself. The normal values given here have been obtained from a wide selection of laboratory and medical sources currently available.

For further information about any test, diagnostic procedure, or disease, consult your local librarian, who can suggest books that offer detailed information on any of these topics.

SECTION 1:
ABBREVIATIONS

A

AB: abortion; absorptiometry

ABG: arterial blood gas (analysis)

ABP: arterial blood pressure

ACG: angiocardiography; apexcardiogram

ACLS: advanced cardiac life support

ACP: acid phosphatase

ACTH: adrenocorticotropic hormone

ACUS: atypical cells of undetermined significance

AD: Alzheimer's disease

ADC: AIDS dementia complex

ADD: attention deficit disorder

ADNase: antideoxyribonuclease

AEP: average evoked potential

AF: amniotic fluid; atrial fibrillation

AFB: acid-fast bacilli

A/G ratio: albumin/globulin ratio

AGG: agammaglobulinemia

AGL: acute granulocytic leukemia

a-HBD: a-hydroxybutyric dehydrogenase

AHD: atherosclerotic heart disease

AHM: ambulatory Holter monitoring

AIDS: acquired immunodeficiency syndrome

ALA: aminolevulinic acid

Alb: albumin

Alc: alcohol

Ald: aldolase

Ald assay: aldolase assay

ALL: acute lymphocytic (lymphoblastic) leukemia

ALP: alkaline phosphatase

ALS: amyotrophic lateral sclerosis

AMI: acute myocardial infarction

AML: acute myelocytic leukemia

ANA: antinuclear antibody

Anti-DNase B: antideoxyribonuclease B

Anti-DS-DNA: anti-double-stranded deoxyribonucleic acid

Anti-ENA: anti-extractable nuclear antigen

ANUG: acute necrotizing ulcerative gingivitis

APPY: appendectomy

APTT: activated partial thromboplastin time

A&P: anterior and posterior; auscultation and percussion

ARC: AIDS-related complex

ARD: AIDS-related disease

ARDS: acute respiratory distress syndrome; adult respiratory distress syndrome

ARF: acute renal failure; acute respiratory failure

ARS: AIDS-related syndrome

ARS-A: arylsulfatase-A

As: arsenic

ASH: antistreptococcal hyaluronidase

ASHD: arteriosclerotic heart disease

ASLO: antistreptolysin-O

AST: aspartate aminotransferase

ATA: antithyroglobulin antibody

ATL: adult T-cell leukemia; adult T-cell lymphoma

AU: Australian antigen

AV: arteriovenous

AV block: atrioventricular block

AWMI: anterior wall myocardial infarction

AZ: Aschheim-Zondek (test)

B

BAC: blood alcohol concentration

BAO: basal acid output

BBB: bundle branch block

BCG: Bacillus Calmette-Guérin

BCLS: basic cardiac life support

BE: bacterial endocarditis; barium enema; base excess

Be: beryllium

BEI: butanol-extractable iodine

BG: blood gases

bili: bilirubin

bl cult: blood culture

bleed and CT: bleeding and clotting time

BM: bowel movement

B2M: beta-2 microglobulin

BMR: basal metabolic rate

BMT: bone marrow transplantation

BP: blood pressure

BPH: benign prostatic hypertrophy (hyperplasia)

BSA: body surface area

BSST: breast stimulation stress test

BTB: breakthrough bleeding

BUN: blood urea nitrogen

BX: biopsy

C

C: Celsius

Ca: calcium; cancer

CA: cardiac arrest; coccidioidomycosis antibody

CAD: coronary artery disease

cAMP: cyclic adenosine monophosphate

CAPD: continuous ambulatory peritoneal dialysis

CAT: computerized axial tomography

CBBB: complete bundle branch block

CCF: congestive cardiac failure

CCPD: continuous cycling peritoneal dialysis

CD4 cell: CD4 (T4) cell count

CEA: carcinoembryonic antigen

CENOG: computerized electroneuro-ophthalmogram

ceph-floc: cephalin-cholesterol flocculation

CF: cystic fibrosis

CFS: chronic fatigue syndrome

CHB: complete heart block

CHD: congenital heart disease

CHF: congestive heart failure

CHO: carbohydrate

chol: cholesterol

CHR: cercarianhullenreaktion

CI: color index

C_l**:** lung compliance (test)

CIN: chronic interstitial nephritis; cervical intraepithelial neoplasia

Cl: chloride

CMG: cystometrogram

CML: chronic myelogenous leukemia

CMV: cytomegalovirus

CNS: central nervous system

CO: cardiac output

CO₂: carbon dioxide

COAD: chronic obstructive airway disease

coag: coagulation

COPD: chronic obstructive pulmonary disease

CP: cor pulmonale; cerebral palsy

CPH: chronic persistent hepatitis

CPK: creatinine phosphokinase

CPR: cardiopulmonary resuscitation

CPT: current procedural terminology

creat: creatinine

CRF: chronic renal failure; chronic respiratory failure

CRP: C-reactive protein

CRS: Chinese restaurant syndrome

CSF: cerebrospinal fluid

CST: contraction stress test

CT: clotting time

CTS: carpal tunnel syndrome

Cu: copper

cult: culture

CVA: cerebrovascular accident

CVD: cardiovascular disease

CVP: central venous pressure

CVRD: cardiovascular renal disease

CVS: chorionic villi sampling

D

D&C: dilation and curettage

defib: defibrillate, defibrillator

DFA-TP: direct fluorescent antibody staining for Treponema pallidum

DHA: dehydroepiandrosterone

DI: diabetes insipidus

DIC: disseminated intravascular coagulation

diff: differential

DM: diabetes mellitus

DNA: deoxyribonucleic acid

DNCB: dinitrochlorobenzene

DOA: dead on arrival

DSA: digital subtraction angiography

DSE: digital subtraction echocardiogram

DST: dexamethasone suppression test

DT: delirium tremens

DUB: dysfunctional uterine bleeding

DUF: doppler ultrasonic flowmeter

D$_x$: diagnosis

E

EAB: elective abortion

EBV: Epstein-Barr virus

ECC: external cardiac compression

ECCE: extracapsular cataract extraction

ECG: electrocardiogram

EchoEEG: echoencephalogram

ECIB: extracorporeal irradiation of blood

ECT: electroconvulsive therapy

EEG: electroencephalogram

EES: endocardial electrical stimulation

EF: ejection fraction

EGD: esophagogastroduodenoscopy

EKG: electrocardiogram

ELISA: enzyme-linked immunosorbent assay

EMG: electromyogram

EPM: evoked potential monitoring

EPS: electrophysiologic study

ER: estrogen receptor

ERBD: endoscopic retrograde biliary drainage

ERCP: endoscopic retrograde cholangiopancreatography

ERUS: endorectal ultrasound

ESR: erythrocyte sedimentation rate

ESRD: end-stage renal disease

EST: electroshock therapy; exercise stress testing

ESWL: extracorporeal shock wave lithotripsy

etiol: etiology

EVS: endoscopic variceal sclerotherapy

F

F: Fahrenheit

FBS: fasting blood sugar

FDP: fibrin degradation products

Fe: iron

FeBC: iron-binding capacity

femto: metric measurement = 10^{15}

FEV: forced expiratory volume (timed)

FFA: free fatty acid

FIA: fluorescent immunoassay

fib: fibrillation

FIGLU: formiminoglutamic acid

FN: false negative

FP: false positive

FSH: follicle-stimulating hormone

FSH & LH: follicle-stimulating hormone and luteinizing hormone (pituitary gonadotropins)

FSP: fibrin split products

FTA-ABS: fluorescent treponemal antibody absorption

FUO: fever of unknown origin

FXS: fragile X syndrome

G

GA: gastric analysis

gal: galactose

GBIA: Guthrie bacterial inhibition assay

GB series: gallbladder series

GC: gas chromatography; gonococcus; gonorrhea

GER: gastroesophageal reflux

GF-BAO: gastric fluid, basal acid output

GG: gammaglobulin

GGT: gamma-glutamyl transferase

GGTP: gamma-glutamyl transpeptidase

GHD: growth hormone deficiency

GIFT: gamete intrafallopian transfer

GI series: gastrointestinal series

GnRH: gonadotropin-releasing hormone

GnST: gonadotropin stimulation test

G-6-PD or G6PD: glucose-6-phosphate-dehydrogenase

GTT: glucose tolerance test

GU: genitourinary; gastric ulcer

G. vaginalis: Gardnerella vaginalis

H

HAA: hepatitis-associated antigen

HAAg: hepatitis A antigen

HAS: hypertensive arteriosclerosis

HAV: hepatitis A virus

HB: heart block

HbA$_{1c}$: hemoglobin, glycosylated

HbA$_2$: hemoglobin A$_2$

HBAg: hepatitis B antigen

HB$_c$Ab: hepatitis B core antibody

HB$_c$Ag: hepatitis B core antigen

HBD: hydroxybutyric dehydrogenase

HbF: fetal hemoglobin; hemoglobin F

HBIG: hepatitis B immunoglobulin

HBO: hyperbaric oxygen

HBV: hepatitis B virus

HCG: human chorionic gonadotropin

HCL: hairy-cell leukemia

HCO$_3$: bicarbonate

H$_2$CO$_3$: carbonic acid

HCS: human chorionic somatotropin

Hct: hematocrit

HDLC: high density lipoprotein cholesterol

H-flu: Haemophilus influenza

Hgb: hemoglobin

HGH: human growth hormone

5-HIAA: 5-hydroxyindoleacetic acid

HIT: hemagglutination inhibition test

HIV: human immunodeficiency virus

HIV-Ab: HIV antibody

HIV-Ag: HIV antigen

HIVIG: anti-HIV immune serum globulin

HL-A: human leukocyte locus A antigen

HLP: hairy leukoplakia

Hp: haptoglobin

HPL: human placental lactogen

HPV: human papillomavirus

HSV$_1$: herpes simplex virus type 1

HSV$_2$: herpes simplex virus type 2

HT: hypertension

HTLV: human T-lymphotropic virus

HVA: homovanillic acid

HVE: high voltage electrophoresis

HZV: herpes zoster virus

I

IADSA: intra-arterial digital subtraction angiography

IAGT: indirect antiglobulin test (indirect Coomb's test)

IBC: iron-binding capacity

IC: intravascular coagulation

ICDH: isocitric dehydrogenase

ICP: intracranial pressure

ICT: indirect Coomb's test

IDDM: insulin-dependent diabetes mellitus

IF: intrinsic factor

IFA: immunofluorescent antibody

IG: immunoglobulin

IH: infectious hepatitis

IHD: ischemic heart disease

IICP: increased intracranial pressure

IM: intramuscular

immunol: immunology

incompat: incompatible

infect: infection

IOP: intraocular pressure

IPP: inflatable penile prosthesis

IPPA: inspection, palpation, percussion, auscultation

IPPB: intermittent positive pressure breathing

IRDS: infant respiratory distress syndrome

I sat %: iron saturation, percent

isoenz: isoenzyme

ITP: idiopathic thrombocytopenic purpura

I & A: irrigation and aspiration

I & D: incision and drainage

I & O: intake and output

IU: international unit

IUD: intrauterine device

IV: intravenous

IVF: in-vitro fertilization

IVGTT: intravenous glucose tolerance test

IVP: intravenous pyelogram

J

jaund: jaundice

JRA: juvenile rheumatoid arthritis

JROM: joint range of motion

K

K: potassium

KA: ketoacidosis

KS: ketosteroids

17-KS: 17-ketosteroids

KJ: knee jerk

KV: killed virus

KVO: keep vein open

L

LA: lactic acid

LAP: leucine aminopeptidase; leukocyte alkaline phosphatase

LATS: long-acting thyroid stimulating hormone

LAV: lymphadenopathy-associated virus

LBP: low blood pressure

LCL: lymphocytic leukemia

LD: Legionnaire's disease

LDH: lactic dehydrogenase

LDLC: low density lipoprotein cholesterol

LE: lupus erythematosus

LE prep: lupus erythematosus (cell) preparation

LE test: lupus erythematosus (cell) test

LF: latex fixation

LGV: lymphogranuloma venereum

LH: luteinizing hormone

LH-FSH: luteinizing hormone-follicle-stimulating hormone

LHRF: luteinizing hormone releasing factor

LHRH: luteinizing hormone releasing hormone

Li: lithium

LIP: lymphoid interstitial pneumonia

LMP: last menstrual period

LP: lumbar puncture

L/S ratio: lecithin/sphingomyelin ratio

LT: lactose tolerance

LTB: laryngotracheobronchitis

M

MAI: Mycobacterium avium intracellulare

MAbs: monoclonal antibodies

MAO: monoamine oxidase

MAOI: monoamine oxidase inhibitor

MBC: maximum breathing capacity

Mc-Ab: monoclonal antibodies

MCH: mean corpuscular hemoglobin

MCHC: mean corpuscular hemoglobin concentration

MCV: mean corpuscular volume

MDR-TB: multidrug-resistant tuberculosis

metab: metabolism

MF: mycosis fungoides

Mg: magnesium

MG: myasthenia gravis

MHA: microhemagglutination assay

MI: myocardial infarction

MIC antibody: microsomal antibody (thyroid)

MIC/MBC: minimal inhibitory concentration/minimal bactericidal concentration

MMEF: maximum mid-expiratory flow

MMPI: Minnesota Multiphasic Personality Inventory

MNCV: motor nerve conduction velocity

MND: motor neuron disease

MODY: mature onset of diabetes in the young

MRA: magnetic resonance angiography

MRI: magnetic resonance imaging

MS: multiple sclerosis

MTT: mean transit time

MVC: maximum vital capacity

MVP: mitral valve prolapse

MVV: maximal voluntary ventilation

N

N: nitrogen

Na: sodium

NCV: nerve conduction velocity

NGT: nasogastric tube

NGU: nongonococcal urethritis

NH$_3$: ammonia

NH$_4$: ammonium

NIDDM: non-insulin-dependent diabetes mellitus

NMR: nuclear magnetic resonance

NPN: nonprotein nitrogen

NPSG: nocturnal polysomnography

NPT: nocturnal penile tumescence

NSAIDS: nonsteroidal anti-inflammatory drugs

5'N: 5'-nucleotidase

NUG: necrotizing ulcerative gingivitis

O

O$_2$: oxygen

OC: oral contraceptive

O$_2$CT: oxygen concentration

OCT: ornithine carbamoyl transferase

OD: right eye (oculus dexter)

OGTT: oral glucose tolerance test

17-OHCS: 17 hydroxycorticosteroids

OI: opportunistic infection

ORIF: open reduction and internal fixation

OS: left eye (oculus sinister)

OSA: obstructive sleep apnea

O₂Sat: oxygen saturation

O & P: ova and parasites

P

P: phosphorus

PAB: premature atrial beat

PAC: premature atrial contraction

PAH: para-aminohippuric acid

PAIDS: pediatric AIDS

PAP: positive airway pressure

Pap smear: Papanicolaou smear

PAT: paroxysmal atrial tachycardia

PAWP: pulmonary artery wedge pressure

Pb: lead

PBI: protein-bound iodine

PC: phenol coefficient

PCA: patient-controlled analgesia

PCG: phonocardiogram

pCO$_2$ (PaCO$_2$): partial pressure of carbon dioxide

PCOD: polycystic ovarian disease

PCP: Pneumocystis carinii pneumonia

PCR: polymerase chain reaction

PEEP: positive end-expiratory pressure

PEG: pneumoencephalogram

PET: positron emission tomography

PGL: persistent generalized lymphadenopathy

PgRT: progesterone receptor test

pH: hydrogen ion concentration (acidity or alkalinity)

phos: phosphatase

phy: phytohemagglutinin (test)

PID: pelvic inflammatory disease

PKU: phenylketonuria

PMS: premenstrual stress

PNH: paroxysmal nocturnal hemoglobinuria

PO$_2$ (PaO$_2$): partial pressure of oxygen

PO$_4$: phosphate

PPD: purified protein derivative

PPNG: penicillinase-producing Neisseria gonorrhoeae

PRA: plasma renin activity

PSA: prostate-specific antigen

PSC: posterior subcapsular cataract

PSP: phenolsulfophthalein

PSVT: paroxysmal supraventricular tachycardia

PT: prothrombin time; paroxysmal tachycardia

PTCA: percutaneous transluminal coronary angioplasty

PTH: parathyroid hormone

PTT: partial thromboplastin time

P & A: percussion and auscultation

PV: plasma volume

PVC: premature ventricular contraction

PVD: peripheral vascular disease

PWARC: persons with AIDS-related complex

P wave: electrocardiogram

p24: p24 antigen (test)

Q

QC: quality control

QNS: quantity not sufficient

QRC: qualitative radiocardiography

QRS: QRS complex (electrocardiogram)

Q suff.: quantum sufficit (adequate quantity)

R

R: roentgen

RA: rheumatoid arthritis

rad: radiation absorbed dose

RAI: radioactive iodine

RAST: radioallergosorbent test

RBC: red blood cell

RCC: red cell count

RCV: red cell volume

RDS: respiratory distress syndrome

rem: roentgen equivalent, man

REM: rapid eye movement

RF: rheumatoid factor

Rh: Rhesus factor

RHD: rheumatic heart disease

RI: refractive index

RIA: radioimmunoassay

RICE: rest, ice, compression, elevation

RLF: retrolental fibroplasia

RLQ: right lower quadrant

RNA: ribonucleic acid

RNP: ribonucleoprotein

ROM: range of motion

ROMI: rule out myocardial infarction

RPG: retrograde pyelogram

RS: respiratory syncytial

RT: radiation therapy

RV: rubella virus; residual volume

S

SA: sinus arrhythmia

SAS: sleep apnea syndrome

SBE: subacute bacterial endocarditis

SBT: simplate bleeding time

SC: subcutaneous

SF: spinal fluid

SG: specific gravity

SGOT: serum glutamic oxaloacetic transaminase

SH: serum hepatitis

SIDS: sudden infant death syndrome

SIG: sigmoidoscopy

SIV: simian immunodeficiency virus

SLE: systemic lupus erythematosus

SMA: sequential multiple analysis

SMD: senile macular degeneration

SOB: short of breath

spec: specimen; speculum

sp gr: specific gravity

SSS: sick sinus syndrome

ST: sinus tachycardia

Staph: Staphylococcus

STD: sexually transmitted disease

strep: Streptococcus

stress ECG: stress electrocardiogram

ST seg: ST segment (electrocardiogram)

SUD: sudden unexpected death

T

T$_3$: triiodothyronine

T$_3$ resin uptake: triiodothyronine resin uptake

T$_4$: thyroxine

TA: toxoplasma antibodies

TA-AIDS: transfusion-associated AIDS

TAB: therapeutic abortion

Tach: tachycardia

TAO: thromboangiitis obliterans

TB: tuberculosis

TBC: tuberculosis; thyroid-binding capacity

TBG: thyroxine-binding globulin

TBI: total body irradiation

TC: total cholesterol

T & C: type and cross-match

TCMI: T-cell mediated immunity

TCT: thrombin clotting time

TDF: tetralogy of Fallot

TDM: therapeutic drug monitoring

TdT: terminal deoxynucleotidyl transferase

TDT: tumor doubling time

TFA: total fatty acids

TG: triglyceride

TGT: thromboplastin generation test time

THR: total hip replacement

TIA: transient ischemic attack

TIBC: total iron-binding capacity

TLC: total lung capacity

TMA: thyroid microsomal antibody

TMJD: temporomandibular joint dysfunction

TMST: treadmill stress test

TNF: tumor necrosis factor

TOF: tetralogy of Fallot

Tot prot or TP: total proteins

TP: thrombocytopenic purpura

TPR: temperature, pulse, respiration

TRUS: transrectal ultrasonography

TSH: thyroid-stimulating hormone

TSI: thyroid-stimulating immunoglobulin

TSS: toxic shock syndrome

TT: thrombin time

TTNB: transient tachypnea of the newborn. See: Infant respiratory distress syndrome (IRDS).

TUA: tubo-ovarian abscess

TV: total volume

T wave: T wave (electrocardiogram)

U

UA: uric acid

UB: urinary bilinogen

UCl: urinary clearance

UO: unknown origin

UPEP: urinary protein electrophoresis

URI: upper respiratory infection

urine spec: urine specimen

US: ultrasound

UTI: urinary tract infection

UVB$_{12}$BC: unsaturated vitamin B$_{12}$ binding capacity

V

v: vein

v: venereal

V: ventilation

vacc: vaccination; vaccine

VC: vital capacity

VCG: vectorcardiogram

VDRL test: Venereal Disease Research Laboratory test

V$_e$: minute ventilation

vect: vector

vent scan: ventilation scan

VEP: visual evoked potential

VF: ventricular fibrillation; visual field

VG: ventricular gallop

VH: viral hepatitis

visc: viscous; viscosity

vit: vitamin

vit A tol: vitamin A tolerance

VLDL: very low density lipoprotein

VMA: 3-methoxy-4-hydroxymandelic acid (also known as vanillylmandelic acid)

V/Q ratio: test of perfusion

VRI: viral respiratory infection

V$_T$: tidal volume

VT: venous thrombosis

V tach: ventricular tachycardia

V-veins: varicose veins

VZV: varicella zoster virus

W

WB: Western blot

WBC: white blood cell

Wd cult: wound culture

WK: Wernicke-Korsakoff syndrome

X

X match: crossmatch

XRT: radiation therapy

Z

ZIFT: zygote intrafallopian tube transfer

Zn: zinc

ZnSO$_4$ turb: zinc sulfate turbidity

SECTION 2:
DEFINITIONS

A

Abdominal aortography: an X-ray study of the abdominal aorta and nearby blood vessels after either injection of contrast medium directly into the aorta or various other injection techniques.

Abortion: miscarriage; loss of pregnancy that may be spontaneous or induced by medication or surgery.

Abscess: an internal or external localized area of infection, usually caused by bacteria, consisting of a pus-filled cavity surrounded by an area of inflamed tissue.

Absorptiometry: a diagnostic procedure done on a person's wrist or spine to determine bone density. Low bone density may indicate bone diseases such as osteoporosis.

Acetoacetic acid: a ketone body produced by metabolic disease or disturbance; also known as diacetic acid.
Normal value: in blood, negative; in urine, negative.

Acetone: a ketone body produced by metabolic disease or disturbance.
Normal value: in blood, negative; in urine, negative.

Acid-fast bacilli: an organism that has special staining characteristics; one such bacillus causes tuberculosis.

Acid phosphatase: an enzyme that is primarily present in the prostate gland. Smaller amounts are found in blood cells and constituents, bone, and other body organs. Elevated levels may signify prostate cancer and various other diseases.
Normal values in blood: 0.5-2 Bodansky units/dL.

Acidosis: an abnormal acid condition of the blood.

Aciduria: abnormally acid urine.

Acquired immunodeficiency syndrome (AIDS): an abnormal condition of the immune system diagnosed by one or more indicator diseases and by laboratory proof of HIV infection.

Acromegaly: a condition caused by excessive secretion of pituitary growth hormone. Abnormal cartilage growth causes enlargement of hands, feet, facial features and, in children, exaggerated height.

Activated partial thromboplastin time (APTT): a blood test done to screen for coagulation (blood clotting) disorders, and to determine the adequacy of various clotting factors.
Normal values: in venous blood 32-51 sec.

Acute granulocytic leukemia: a cancerous disease of blood, in which there is an increase of white (granulocyte) blood cells.

Acute lymphocytic leukemia: a cancerous blood disease in which there is an increase of white (lymphocyte) blood cells.

Acute myelocytic leukemia: a cancerous blood disease in which there is an increase of white (myelocyte) blood cells.

Acute myocardial infarct: a heart attack (damaged heart muscle due to inadequate blood supply).

Acute necrotizing (pseudomembranous) enterocolitis: a serious, sometimes fatal, inflammatory bowel disease that may follow intestinal surgery or administration of certain antibiotics. Bacterial overgrowth causes formation of raised, yellowish, membrane-like plaques on intestinal tissues.

Acute necrotizing ulcerative gingivitis, Vincent's disease: a serious disease of the gums causing ulcers and destruction of the gums and surrounding tissues.

Acute renal failure: a condition in which the kidneys suddenly cease to produce urine and to filter waste products from the blood. Cessation may be partial or total.

Acute respiratory distress syndrome: sudden, severe failure of the lungs to exchange oxygen and carbon dioxide.

Acute respiratory failure: sudden inability of the lungs to carry out their functions in exchanging oxygen and carbon dioxide.

Addis count: a test done on urine to detect kidney disease.
  Normal values: in urine after 12-hr collection:
      white blood cells (WBC) and epithelial cells, 1,800,000;
      red blood cells (RBC), 500,000;
      hyaline casts, 0-5,000.

Addison's disease: an illness caused by insufficient production of hormones in the outer section of the adrenal glands, one situated above each kidney. Hormone deficiency causes fluid and salt loss from the body. Symptoms include fatigue, weight loss, skin darkening, muscle weakness, low blood pressure, vomiting, and diarrhea.

Adrenaline: see Epinephrine

Adrenocorticotropic hormone (ACTH): a pituitary hormone that stimulates the adrenal cortex.

Adrenocorticotropic hormone (ACTH) stimulation test: see Corticotropin (ACTH) response test.

Adult T cell leukemia (lymphoma): cancer of the blood that affects the lymph glands, liver, spleen, and causes various other symptoms.

Advanced life support: maintaining a person's vital functions with the aid of complex equipment.

Aerobic organism (aerobe): a microorganism that requires atmospheric oxygen in order to grow.

Agammaglobulinemia: a deficiency of antibodies in blood, which reduces a person's ability to ward off infection.

Agar: a substance used in the laboratory to culture microorganisms.

Agglutination: a process in which cells suspended in fluid clump together and become visible to the naked eye.

Agglutinins: antibodies that produce agglutination (clumping) of various types of cells.

Agglutinogen: an antigen that stimulates the production of agglutinins.

AIDS dementia complex: brain deterioration, caused by the AIDS virus, leading to difficulty in thinking or managing daily activities.

AIDS-related complex (ARC): a combination of two or more designated conditions lasting for three or more months that indicate the probable onset of AIDS at a future time.

AIDS-related diseases: infections and other abnormalities associated with HIV infection.

Albumin: a protein elevated in blood (in the presence of kidney or various other diseases); in cerebral spinal fluid (CSF) (in the presence of infection or other diseases); or in urine (found in appreciable amounts only in the presence of kidney or various other diseases).
> *Normal values:* in serum, 3.2-5.6 g/dL; in CSF, 10-30 mg/dL;
> in random urine, negative to trace, qualitative;
> in urine 24-hr collection, negative or 10-100 mg, quantitative.

Albumin : Globulin ratio: the ratio of albumin to globulin, altered in certain pathological conditions such as multiple myeloma.
Normal values:
in plasma or serum, 1.3 : 3.0;
in CSF, 1.6 : 2.2.

Alcohol: an intoxicating agent present in blood after ingestion.
Normal value: in serum or whole blood, negative.

Aldolase assay: a test to determine blood levels of aldolase, an enzyme that converts sugar to energy in the muscles. It is elevated in various conditions, including liver necrosis, skeletal muscle disease, granulocytic leukemia, and muscular dystrophy.
Normal values: in serum, 0-11 mIU/mL (varies by laboratory method).

Aldosterone: a mineralocorticoid substance produced in the adrenal cortex, which regulates water reabsorption and several other conditions.
Normal values: in serum, 3-10 ng/dL; may go higher in the standing patient.

Aliquot: a small, measured sample of body or other fluid.

Alkaline phosphatase: a blood test used to measure an enzyme to determine the presence of skeletal diseases and certain types of liver diseases.
Normal values:
in men, 90-239 U/L;
in women under 45, 76-196 U/L;
in women over 45, 87-250 U/L;
in children, levels are up to 3 times those of adults.

Alkalosis: disruption of the body's acid-base balance by an excessive increase in the blood alkali level. Acid loss may result from severe vomiting or ingestion of large amounts of antacids or diuretics.

Alkapton bodies: a class of substances, especially homogentisic acid, present in urine in alkaptonuria, a rare metabolic disease.
Normal value: negative.

Allergen: a substance capable of causing allergy in a susceptible person.

Allergy: hypersensitivity to a specific substance.

Alpha-fetoprotein: see α_1-Fetoprotein.

Alzheimer's disease: a degenerative disease of the brain, usually occurring in middle-aged or elderly people, characterized by loss of memory and progressive mental deterioration.

Ambulatory Holter monitoring: a device worn round the clock in order to monitor and diagnose heart actions and irregularities.

Ameba (amoeba): a one-celled protozoan organism that moves via projections called pseudopods.

Amebiasis: an infection caused by amebas; also called amebic dysentery.

Amenorrhea: the absence of menstruation.

Amino acid: a component of body protein.

α-Amino acid nitrogen: a substance measured in urine to diagnose various metabolic disturbances.
Normal values: in urine after 24-hr collection, 50-200 mg.

Aminoaciduria: an excessive amount of one or more amino acids in the urine.

α-Amino-n-butyric acid: a substance present in the blood of heavy alcohol drinkers. *Normal value:* negative.

Aminoglycoside serum assay: a blood test done to make sure that antibiotic drugs are administered in dosages that maintain therapeutic blood levels.

β-Aminolevulinic acid: a protein product of metabolism, measured in blood to diagnose lead poisoning or porphyria (a blood disease) or in urine to diagnose lead poisoning.
Normal values:
in serum, 0.01-0.03 mL/dL;
in random urine,
in adults, 0.1-0.6 mg/dL;
in children, 0.5 mg/dL;
in urine after 24-hr collection, 1.3-7.0 mg.

Ammonia: a substance produced by bacterial activity in the intestine; measured in blood to determine adequate liver function in converting ammonia into urea, a substance secreted by the kidneys. Serum ammonia levels rise in liver disease and are useful in diagnosing impending or established hepatic coma, as well as for monitoring treatment. Elevated serum ammonia levels may also be helpful in diagnosing Reye's syndrome.
Normal values:
in venous or arterial blood, 40-70 μg/100 mL;
in plasma, 20-150 μg/dL (by diffusion method).

Ammonia nitrogen: a substance measured in urine to determine the body's acid-base balance and nitrogen balance.
Normal values:
in random urine, 35-70 μg/dL;
in urine after 24-hr collection, 20-70 mEq; 500-1200 mg.

Amniocentesis: insertion of a needle through the abdomen into a pregnant woman's uterus (womb) to obtain a sample of amniotic fluid (the fluid that surrounds the fetus) for detection of the sex and various genetic factors or diseases of the unborn child.

Amniotic fluid (AF): liquid contained in the amnion, or amniotic sac, which surrounds the fetus in the placenta inside the womb.

Amniotic fluid, absorbance difference at 450 nm: a test done on AF via spectrophotometry to detect fetal blood abnormalities in early or late pregnancy.
Normal values:
> early pregnancy, less than 0.05 optical density difference (ODD);
> at term, less than 0.02 ODD.

Amniotic fluid, appearance: a test for normal visual appearance of the AF in early or late pregnancy.
Normal values:
> early pregnancy (before 28 weeks), clear;
> at term, clear or slightly opalescent.

Amniotic fluid, bilirubin: a test done on AF to detect fetal abnormalities, such as hemolytic disease, in early or late pregnancy.
Normal values:
> early pregnancy, less than 0.075 mg/dL;
> at term, less than 0.025 mg/dL.

Amniotic fluid, chloride: a test done on AF to detect fetal problems in early or late pregnancy.
Normal values:
> early pregnancy, about equal to serum chloride;
> at term, generally lower than serum chloride.

Amniotic fluid, creatinine: a test done on AF to determine the age of the fetus.
Normal values:
> early pregnancy, 0.8-1.1 mg/dL;
> at term, 1.8-4.4 mg/dL, usually more than 2.0 mg/dl.

Amniotic fluid, cytologic staining (Nile blue sulfate): a count of fat-staining cells in a sample of AF, done to determine the age of the fetus.
Normal values:
early pregnancy, less than 2% of total cells;
at term, greater than 20% or more of total cells.

Amniotic fluid, estriol: a test done on AF to detect fetal abnormalities, such as fetoplacental depression, in early or late pregnancy.
Normal values:
early pregnancy, less than 10 µg/dL;
at term, greater than 60 µg/dL.

Amniotic fluid, lecithin/sphingomyelin ratio: the ratio of two components of AF, found to be a predictor of fetal lung maturity.
Normal ratio: 2 : 1 or greater.

Amniotic fluid, osmolality: a test done on AF to detect fetal abnormalities in early or late pregnancy.
Normal values:
early pregnancy, about equal to serum osmolality;
at term, less than 250 mOsm/L.

Amniotic fluid, PCO_2: measurement of the partial pressure of carbon dioxide in AF to detect fetal abnormalities in early or late pregnancy.
Normal values:
early pregnancy, 33-55 mm Hg;
at term, 42-55 mm Hg (increases toward term).

Amniotic fluid, pH: measurement of the acidity or alkalinity of AF, done to detect fetal distress or other fetal abnormalities in early or late pregnancy.
Normal values:
early pregnancy, 7.12-7.38;
at term, 6.91-7.43 (decreases toward term).

49

Amniotic fluid, rapid surfactant test: a test done on AF to detect fetal lung maturity.
Normal value: a complete ring of bubbles persisting 15 min at 1:1 dilution only.

Amniotic fluid, sodium: a test done on AF to detect fetal problems in early or late pregnancy.
Normal values:
early pregnancy, about equal to serum sodium;
at term, about 7-10 mEq/L lower than serum sodium.

Amniotic fluid, total protein: a test done on AF to detect fetal abnormalities in early or late pregnancy.
Normal values:
early pregnancy, 0.60 ± 0.24 g/dL;
at term, 0.26 ± 0.19 g/dL.

Amniotic fluid, urea: a test done on AF to detect fetal problems in early or late pregnancy.
Normal values:
early pregnancy, 18.0 ± 5.9 mg/dL;
at term, 30.3 ± 11.4 mg/dL.

Amniotic fluid, uric acid: a test done on AF to detect fetal problems in early or late pregnancy.
Normal values:
early pregnancy, 3.72 ± 0.96 mg/dL;
at term, 9.9 ± 2.23 mg/dL.

Amniotic fluid, volume: measurement of AF volume to detect fetal abnormalities in early or late pregnancy.
Normal values:
early pregnancy, 450-1200 mL;
at term, 500-1400 mL (increases toward term).

Amylase: an enzyme secreted by the pancreas that is elevated in diseases of the pancreas or salivary glands, kidney problems, and drug ingestion.
Normal values:
in serum, 25-125 mIU/mL;
in urine, 1-17 U/h.

Amyotrophic lateral sclerosis (ALS): a disease marked by gradual deterioration of the motor nerve cells of the lateral columns and anterior horns of the spinal cord, resulting in progressive atrophy of the arms, legs, trunk, and respiratory muscles. Also called Lou Gehrig's Disease.

Anaerobic organism (anaerobe): a microorganism that can grow only in the absence of atmospheric oxygen.

Anaphylaxis: an extreme allergic state that may be fatal if not immediately treated effectively.

Androsterone: a sex hormone secreted by the testes and the adrenal glands.
Normal values: in urine after 24-hour collection:
in men, 2.8-5.0 mg;
in women, 0.8-3.0 mg.

Anergy: absence of reaction to substances that normally provoke a sensitivity response by the body; usually caused by an inadequate immune system.

Anemia: a blood disorder characterized by fewer-than-normal red blood cells (erythrocytes) and a lower-than-normal quantity of hemoglobin.

Aneurysm: a sac formed by dilation of a weakened area in the wall of a blood vessel, generally an artery. When the area ruptures, severe bleeding may result. Aneurysms most commonly occur in the chest, abdomen, and brain.

Angina pectoris: pain in the region of the heart that sometimes radiates down the left arm. Caused by poor blood supply or spasms in the heart's arteries.

Angina, unstable: unpredictable occurrence of pain in the region of the heart, not necessarily in response to exercise.

Angiocardiogram: a radiographic record of the internal structure of the heart and great blood vessels (pulmonary arteries, veins, and aorta) after injection of contrast medium.

Angioechocardiography: a scan of the blood vessels using ultrasound technique to determine abnormalities in these vessels.

Angiogram: an X-ray examination of the blood vessels of the brain (cerebral) or kidneys (renal) after injection of contrast medium.
Normal value: normal structure of all blood vessels visualized.

Angiography: an X-ray examination of the blood vessels after injection of contrast medium.

Ankylosing spondylitis: inflammation and gradual stiffening of the joints in the spine and in nearby structures as a result of chronic progressive arthritis.

Anorexia nervosa: an eating disorder primarily found in adolescent girls or young women, in which the patient refuses to eat or exhibits abnormal eating patterns that if not treated can lead to severe weight loss, malnutrition, and death.

Anterior and posterior: front and back; terms used to describe anatomic positions.

Anterior wall myocardial infarction: a blood clot and lack of blood supply in the major blood vessels located in the anterior portion of the heart.

Antibacterial serum: serum that can kill bacteria or prevent their growth.

Antibiotic, serum killing level test: an immunologic test that determines the drug level in serum at which an antibiotic drug can inhibit the growth of or kill a given infectious microorganism.
Adequate values: serum can be diluted 1 : 8 or more and is still capable of killing the microorganism causing the infection.

Antibody: a protein substance in blood that can kill or render harmless invading material (such as disease-causing microorganisms) that might cause infection or other damage.

Anticoagulant: a substance that prevents or delays clotting of blood cells.

Antideoxyribonuclease: an antibody substance measured in blood to detect streptococcal infection.
Normal values: in serum, titer of less than 1 : 20.

Antideoxyribonuclease B: an antibody that is measured in blood to diagnose diseases such as rheumatic fever or post-streptococcal glomerulonephritis (kidney disease).
Normal values:
    in whole blood:
        small children, 120 U;
        older children and adults, 1.360 U.

Anti-deoxyribonucleic acid (DNA) antibody assay: a test to detect autoantibodies to double-stranded DNA; used to diagnose and monitor diseases such as systemic lupus erythematosus.

Anti-double-stranded deoxyribonucleic acid (DNA): an antibody substance measured in blood to help diagnose the presence, and monitor the progress, of systemic lupus erythematosus.
Normal values: in whole blood, 1.5 U/mL.

Antiextractable nuclear antigen: an antibody substance measured in blood to aid in the diagnosis of rheumatic diseases.
Normal values: in whole blood, negative.

Antigen: a substance in blood capable of inducing the production of antibodies.

Antinuclear antibodies (ANA): antibody substances measured in blood to detect a wide variety of diseases, including connective tissue disease; drug-associated disease; and others involving the liver, intestines, and circulatory system.
Normal values: in serum, titer of less than 1 : 10

Antiseptic: a substance that checks, or prevents, the growth of microorganisms.

Antiserum: serum that has immune properties (contains antibodies).

Antistreptococcal hyaluronidase: an antibody substance measured in blood to detect streptococcal infection.
Normal values: in serum, titer of less than 1 : 256

Antistreptolysin O: a test done on serum to measure streptolysin O, which kills red blood cells. An immune reaction occurs in which antibodies are produced. In turn, the antistreptolysin O titer is elevated.
Normal value: O negative.

Antithyroglobulin antibody: a thyroid autoantibody, present in patients with autoimmune reactions in the thyroid gland.
Normal values: in serum, titer of less than 1 : 32.

Antitoxin: an immune serum that neutralizes or prevents harmful action by a toxin (a poisonous substance produced by disease-causing microorganisms).

Aortoarteriography: an X-ray study, using a series of films of the circulatory system of the abdomen and a portion of the lower extremities after injection of contrast medium through a needle or catheter into an artery or vein in the lower part of the body.

Apexcardiography: a procedure in which a transducer is applied to the apex of the heart (the lowest point of the heart that is also the farthest to the left), to identify abnormal heart sounds in such conditions as heart valve disease or tumor of the heart muscle.

Aphthous ulcers: painful ulcers in the mouth area often associated with HIV disease.

Aplastic anemia: a form of anemia that results from bone marrow damage or destruction. Bleeding from various parts of the body and frequent infections occur with this disorder.

Appendicitis: inflammation of the vermiform appendix, a small appendage of the large intestine in the right lower abdomen; inflammation may be acute or chronic.

Argininosuccinate lyase: an enzyme used to measure liver function.
Normal values: in serum, 0-4 U/dL.

Arrhythmia: an abnormal rhythm of the heart beat.

Arsenic: a toxic substance found in the blood and urine; elevated levels indicate arsenic poisoning.
Normal values:
in blood, 0.2-6.2 µg/dL;
chronic poisoning, 10-50 µg/dL;
acute poisoning, 60-930 µg/dL;
in urine after 24-hr collection, less than 50 µg/d.

Arterial blood gas analysis: a test done on arterial blood to determine gas exchange in the lungs. See Bicarbonate; Oxygen. Carboxyhemoglobin; Methemoglobin. (see also Partial pressure of carbon dioxide; Partial pressure of oxygen; and pH.)

Arterial blood pressure: blood pressure as measured in a major artery.

Arteriography: an X-ray study of the structure of one or more arteries and other nearby blood vessels after injection of contrast medium.

Arteriosclerosis: a group of conditions that causes the walls of the arteries to become thicker and less elastic; also called hardening of the arteries.

Arteriosclerotic heart disease: see: Atherosclerotic heart disease.

Arteriovenous: refers to an artery and a vein.

Arthritis: a disorder in which joints and their supporting tissues become inflamed and often swollen. The many possible causes include aging, infection, and trauma.

Arthrography: an X-ray examination of the knee joint, and sometimes other joints, done under local anesthesia. Dye is injected into the joint to be examined, and X-rays are taken of the area.

Arthroscopy: a procedure, often done under local anesthesia, that allows direct inspection of the interior of a joint and performance of surgery to correct a diagnosed abnormality, such as a torn ligament, joint disease, torn cartilage, or other problem. The procedure is usually done following arthrography.

Arylsulfatase A: an enzyme; a test is done on urine to aid the diagnosis of cancer of the bladder, colon, or rectum and several other conditions.
Normal values:
in men, 1.4-19.3 U/L;
in women, 1.4-11 U/L;
in children, over 1 U/L.

Ascites: excessive fluid build-up in the abdomen resulting from disease of the heart, liver, lungs, kidneys, and other organs.

Ascorbic acid: vitamin C, which is essential for proper body functioning; deficiency causes scurvy.
Normal values:
in plasma, 0.6-2.0 mg/dL;
in whole blood, 0.7-2.0 mg/dL;
in random urine, 1-7 mg/dL;
in urine after 24-hr collection, more than 50 mg/dL.

Ascorbic acid tolerance: a test to determine the extent of ascorbic acid (vitamin C) deficiency. Blood levels are measured following administration of a known amount of ascorbic acid.
Normal values: in plasma, more than 1.6 mg/dL.

Aseptic: sterile.

Aspartate aminotransferase: see Transaminases.

Aspirate: to suction fluid from the body for examination or to reduce excess fluid.

Assay: analysis of a substance

Asymptomatic HIV infection: infection with the AIDS virus without apparent signs or symptoms.

Atelectasis: collapse of all or part of a lung owing to trauma or disease. In newborns, the term signifies failure of the lungs to expand.

Atherosclerosis: a disease in which yellowish fatty plaques form along the inner walls of the arteries; it is the most common form of arteriosclerosis.

Atherosclerotic heart disease: an illness in which the arteries of the heart become thick, harden, and lose elasticity. This eventually slows or stops the flow of blood, depriving tissues of needed blood supply, and may cause angina or a heart attack.

Atomic absorption spectrophotometry: a technique measuring trace elements (i.e., calcium, magnesium, copper) in body fluids.

Atrial fibrillation: a dangerous irregularity of the heart rhythm.

Atrioventricular block: impaired electrical conduction (regulating the heartbeat) between the atria and the ventricles of the heart.

Atrophy: a reduction in the size of a body part owing to illness or other wasting condition.

Attention deficit disorder: a form of mental illness usually diagnosed during childhood. Symptoms include inability to concentrate, pay attention for any length of time, restlessness, and hyperactivity.

Atypical cells of undetermined significance: unusual cells found in laboratory examination whose importance has not been determined in relation to the patient's condition.

Audiometry: a test to measure hearing function.

Auscultation and percussion: listening to the sounds in, and tapping different parts of, the body to determine various functions and abnormalities.

Australian antigen: an antigen often found in the serum of people who have had hepatitis; the blood test for this antigen is used to detect serum hepatitis (type B) and to differentiate type B from type A hepatitis.

Normal value: negative, but sometimes present in otherwise healthy Americans and in many people who live in the Middle East and Asia.

Autoantibody: an antibody that acts like a foreign substance and may react against normal tissues to cause disease.

Autoantigen: an antigen produced by the body that induces antibody production.

Autoclave: a machine that uses pressurized steam to sterilize objects and equipment.

Autogenous vaccine: a vaccine produced by culturing a patient's own bacteria.

Autoimmune disease: a disease in which the body produces an immune response against itself.

Autoimmunity: a condition that occurs when a patient's antibodies attack his or her own body proteins.

Autoinfection: an infection transferred from an infected body part to one or more additional parts.

Autolysis: destruction of cells by body enzymes.

Autopsy: the external and internal examination of the body after death.

Average evoked potential: a test using electricity to detect the responses of certain nerve pathways, to diagnose various nervous diseases.

Avitaminosis: a deficiency state owing to severe lack of essential vitamins.

Azygography: a radiographic examination of the azygos vein system (posterior chest) after injection of contrast medium.

B

B lymphocytes: lymphocytes (lymph cells) that are bone marrow-dependent (originate in the bone marrow) and function as part of the immune system to protect against infection.

Bacillary dysentery: a bacterial infection of the intestinal tract that causes severe diarrhea, fever, abdominal cramps, nausea, and vomiting. Stools may contain blood or pus.

Bacillus Calmette-Guerin: a bovine tubercle microorganism used in a vaccine that protects against tuberculosis.

Bacteremia: contamination of the bloodstream with bacteria; also called blood poisoning.

Bacterial endocarditis: inflammation of the lining of the heart (endocardium) caused by bacteria.

Bacterial sensitivity test: a laboratory procedure to determine which antibiotic drug will most effectively counteract a specific infection.

Bacterial vaginosis: see *Gardnerella* (bacterial vaginosis).

Bactericide: an agent that kills bacteria.

Bacteriology: the science of bacteria.

Bacteriolysins: antibodies that dissolve bacteria when complement (a normal body protein needed for antigen/antibody reaction) is present.

Bacteriophage: a virus that causes disintegration of bacteria.

Bacteriostasis: a condition that inhibits the growth of bacteria without necessarily killing them.

Bacteroides infection: an infection with bacteria of the genus *Bacteroides*, usually mixed with other bacteria. It is most common after surgery or obstruction of the intestinal tract, but may also occur in the tonsillar area or the female genital tract.

Barbiturates: a class of sedative drugs. Barbiturate blood levels are measured in patients who have taken overdoses either accidentally, to abuse drugs, or intentionally, to commit suicide.
Normal values: in serum, plasma or whole blood, negative.

Barium enema: an X-ray study that uses barium sulfate and air as contrast medium to help with visualization of the interior of the colon.

Barium swallow: an X-ray study in which the patient swallows a mixture of barium sulfate and water to aid visualization of the esophagus; done to detect abnormal conditions of the esophagus.

Basal acid output: see Gastric fluid, basal acid output.

Basal metabolic rate (BMR): a measurement of thyroid function, via a breathing test that measures oxygen used and calories spent while the body is at rest.

Base excess: a test of the body's acid-base balance, measured as bicarbonate.
Normal values: in blood, 0 ± 2 mEq/L.

Basic cardiac life support: life-saving aid given when a person's heart stops beating; done by clearing the throat, administering chest thumps, and inflating the chest by breathing into the person's mouth according to a prescribed pattern.

Bedside radiography: an X-ray study performed at the bedside when the patient is too ill to be moved.

Bell's palsy: a form of facial paralysis, usually affecting only one side, that generally clears up within several weeks but may last longer. Cause is unknown.

Bence Jones protein: a protein excreted in urine in the presence of various conditions such as multiple myeloma.
Normal value: negative.

Benign condition: an abnormal condition that is not malignant (i.e., that does not produce death or deterioration).

Benign prostatic hyperplasia: enlargement of the prostate gland in men, resulting in constriction of the urethra that may interfere with urination.

Beriberi: a disease caused by thiamine (vitamin B_1) deficiency in the diet. Severe deficiency may cause nervous system or circulatory problems, including paralysis or heart failure.

Bernstein test: see Perfusion test, acid.

Beryllium: an element not normally present in urine except in very small quantities.
Normal values: urine after 24-hr collection, less than 0.05 µg.

Beta-2-microglobulin: a blood factor measured to assess the progress of HIV infection and certain other diseases.

Bicarbonate: a constituent of carbonic acid; blood levels of bicarbonate provide an index of the body's alkali reserve.
Normal values: in plasma, 23-29 mEq/L.

Bile: a greenish-yellow to golden brown, bitter-tasting fluid produced by the liver to help digest fats.

Bilharziasis: see Schistosomiasis.

Biliary drainage test: a test of bile fluid drawn from the duodenum (the portion of small intestine adjacent to the stomach) to check for white blood cells, cholesterol, crystals, or parasites.

Bilirubin: a substance formed during the breakdown of hemoglobin in the blood; present in urine in conditions such as obstructive disease of the gallbladder or liver disease.
Normal value: in urine, negative.

Biopsy: the surgical removal of body tissue for microscopic examination.

Biplane cerebral angiography: an X-ray study of the blood vessels in the brain after injection of contrast medium, showing the structures from the side (laterally) and front-to-back (anteroposteriorly).

Bleeding and clotting time: two blood tests, generally performed at the same time, to show how rapidly the small blood vessels constrict to stop bleeding, and how effectively the blood's clotting mechanisms are working.
Normal values: bleeding, 3-10 min (depending on method used); clotting, 5-15 min.

Blood: the fluid that carries nutrients and oxygen to and removes wastes from all parts of the body. It also performs many other vital functions. Blood consists primarily of plasma, red blood cells, white blood cells, and platelets.
Average volume: 8-10 pt.

Blood alcohol concentration: the amount of alcohol in the blood at any time. A person with a blood alcohol concentration of 0.06-0.9 generally is considered "impaired;" a person with a blood alcohol concentration of 1.0 or over generally is considered "intoxicated." Legal concentrations vary from state to state.

Blood culture: the incubation of a blood sample in nutrient material to determine the growth and type of infection-causing microorganisms.

Blood gases: gases dissolved in the blood that maintain its acid-base balance. See also Partial pressure of oxygen; Partial pressure of carbon dioxide; pH.

Blood, occult: small amounts of blood found either in the feces when an abnormality is present somewhere in the gastrointestinal tract; or in the urine in disease of the kidney or urinary tract, or following trauma. Used to detect injury or diseases such as cancer, anemia, and infection.
Normal values: in feces or uring, negative.

Blood pressure: the pressure of the circulating blood against the walls of the blood vessels. Pressure is highest during systole, the phase during which the heart contracts and forces blood into the arteries. Pressure is lowest during diastole, when the heart muscle relaxes. Average pressure may be measured in millimeters of mercury (mm Hg) with an instrument called a sphygmomanometer. A pressure of 120 (systolic) over 80 (diastolic) mm Hg is considered normal. Normal blood pressure varies from one person to another depending on such factors as age, activity, weight, and health. Women tend to have somewhat lower blood pressures than men.

Blood-synovial fluid glucose difference: see Synovial fluid-blood glucose difference.

Blood type: the type and subtype of an individual's blood; specified as A, B, AB, or O; Rh-negative or Rh-positive; and including a number of subtypes. It is important to determine the blood type when a woman is pregnant or when a patient needs a transfusion in order to avoid a dangerous reaction with an incompatible type.

Blood urea nitrogen: see Urea nitrogen.

Blood volume: a measure of a patient's total blood volume.
Normal values:
for whole blood:
in men, 69 mL/kg;
in women, 65 mL/kg.

Body surface area: a calculation based on a person's height and weight, used to determine the appropriate amount of food, fluid, and medication as needed in various circumstances.

Bone densitometry: a radiographic technique used to measure the density of bone, to assess bone structure and strength, and to diagnose such conditions as osteoporosis.

Bone marrow aspiration: removal of bone marrow from the breast bone or hip bone by aspiration through a needle. The blood cells produced by the bone marrow are evaluated as to number, appearance, development, and presence of infection. Done when leukemia, anemia, or other disease affecting the bone marrow is suspected.
Normal values: in bone marrow some 15 different types of cells in given numbers and stages of maturation, as evaluated by a hematologist (blood specialist).

Bone marrow transplantation: replacement of diseased bone marrow (the soft fatty tissues inside bone that produce blood cells) with a graft of a donor's healthy bone marrow; may be done following total body irradiation to prevent rejection of the graft.

Bone scan: a radiographic examination of bone following injection of a radioactive substance into a vein. A scintillating camera (scanner) is used to visualize the bone structure being examined.

Bone X-ray: an X-ray study of bone to determine whether fracture or disease is present.

Botulism: a rarely occurring type of food poisoning caused by the organism *Clostridium botulinum.*

Bradycardia: an abnormally slow heart rate, usually less than 60 beats per minute.

Brain scan: a scan of the brain after injection of radioactive material into a vein. An increased concentration of radioactive material in a given area indicates pathology. The test is done twice; immediately after the injection and again 24 hours later.

Breakthrough bleeding: intermittent spotting that may occur in women who have low levels of estrogen, who use estrogen and progestogen (another female hormone) after menopause, or who have various abnormalities of their reproductive system.

Breast stimulation stress test: a test in which a pregnant woman's breasts are stimulated to contract the womb. During contractions, fetal well-being is assessed by recording and evaluating the fetal heart rate.

Broad-spectrum antibiotic: an antibiotic drug that is effective against a wide range of disease-causing microorganisms.

Bromides: a chemical class found in over-the-counter sedative medications and in some prescription drugs. Blood levels are measured to detect toxicity.
    Normal values: in serum, negative.
    Therapeutic levels: in serum, 0.5 mg/dL.

Bronchogram: a radiographic record of the bronchi and bronchioles after injection of contrast medium.

Bronchoscopy: examination of the bronchi by direct visualization through a bronchoscope, to diagnose abnormalities. The scope may be inserted through the mouth or directly into the trachea via a tracheostomy (surgical opening in the trachea).

Brucella agglutinins: antibodies elevated in blood of patients with brucellosis.
Normal values: in serum, titer of less than 1 : 80.

Buccal smear: cells scraped from the inside of the cheek to detect abnormalities of sexual development.
Normal values:
> *men*, 46 chromosomes, including one X and one Y, no Barr body; *women*, 46 chromosomes, including two X chromosomes, one of which appears as a Barr body.

Buffer: a substance that reduces or prevents excess acid or alkali in the body.

Bulimia: an eating disorder characterized by greatly increased eating (binges), alternating with periods of purging (laxative abuse, vomiting, and greatly reduced eating).

Bundle branch block: ineffectual or no trans-mission of the electrical impulses (governing the heart beat) from the heart's atrium to the ventricle.

Burkitt's lymphoma: a cancerous illness that may affect the ovaries, abdominal lymph nodes, or bones of the face.

C

Calcitonin (thyrocalcitonin): a thyroid hormone measured in blood to detect certain types of cancers. The test is done using a radioimmunoassay technique.

Normal values:

in men (basal), equal or less than 0.155 ng/mL;
women (basal), equal or less than 0.105 ng/mL.

Calcium: a mineral in blood essential for a number of biochemical functions, including transmission of nerve impulses and muscle contractions. It is found in abnormal levels in CSF in the presence of infections such as tuberculous meningitis.

Normal values:

in serum, 9.0-11.0 mg/dL;
in CSF, 2.1-2.6 mEq/L.

Calcium, qualitative: an estimate of the level of calcium in urine, decreased in glandular and nutritional deficiency, increased in patients taking certain diuretic drugs and in some other conditions.

Normal value: 1 + turbidity.

Calcium, quantitative: a measurement of calcium levels in urine, decreased in glandular or nutritional deficiency.

Normal values:

in urine after 24-hr collection:
average diet, 100-250 mg;
low-calcium diet, less than 150 mg;
high-calcium diet, 250-300 mg;
toxic, more than 15 µg/mL.

Caloric test: a test of the inner ear in which hot water or ice is instilled in the ear and eye movements are observed; performed on patients with ear disease or injury or those with symptoms of dizziness or fainting.

Normal values: eye movement toward the site of hot water instillation, away from the site of ice water instillation

Candida albicans: an organism normally present in various body parts (mouth, vagina, intestinal tract) but that may cause infection in patients who have chronic debilitating diseases or HIV infection.

Candidiasis: a sexually transmitted disease (infection), caused by the organism *Candida albicans* that causes a variety of genital and other symptoms.

Capillary fragility test: a test to measure the fragility of small blood vessels near the skin; done with a blood pressure cuff. Fragility of these vessels is indicative of various blood vessel diseases.

Carbohydrates: a class of organic compounds of carbon combined with hydrogen and oxygen, the latter two in the same proportion as in water. The class includes sugars, starches, and cellulose.

Carbon dioxide combining power: a blood test that measures the carbon dioxide absorbed at a given pressure and temperature; done in respiratory and other problems. *Normal values:* in venous plasma or serum, 24-30 mmol/L; 50-58 vol%

Carbon dioxide content: a measurement of carbonic acid and bicarbonate in blood, plasma, or serum; done in respiratory problems.

Normal values:
in whole blood, 19-24 mmol/L;
in arterial plasma or serum, 21-28 mmol/L;
in venous whole blood, 22-26 mmol/L;
in venous plasma or serum, 24-30 mmol/L.

Carbonic acid: an acid that results from dissolving carbon dioxide in water; blood levels are measured to determine respiratory function.
Normal values:
in arterial whole blood, 1.05-1.45 mmol/L;
in venous plasma, 1.02-1.38 mmol/L.

Carboxyhemoglobin: a compound of carbon monoxide and hemoglobin. Carbon monoxide poisoning is detected by measuring the capacity of the heme portion of the hemoglobin (Hgb) molecule to combine with carbon monoxide.
Normal values: in whole blood:
in suburban nonsmokers, less than 1.5% saturation of Hgb;
in smokers, 1.5-5.0%; in heavy smokers, 5.0-9.0%.

Carcinoembryonic antigen: an antigen measured in serum and sometimes other body fluids to detect the presence or recurrence of cancer in such sites as the colon, pancreas, lung, breast, or prostate.
Normal values:
in serum, less than 2 ng/mL; in pregnant women, normal adults, and infants, very small quantities

Cardiac arrest: cessation of the heart beat.

Cardiac catheterization: a diagnostic procedure that involves inserting a catheter into a vein or artery and advancing it under fluoroscopic guidance into the blood vessels or chambers of the heart. Contrast medium is injected to aid in visualization, and blood samples and pressure readings may be taken at different stages.

Cardiac output: the heart's capacity to pump blood.

Cardiac rehabilitation: a process that helps a person who has had a heart attack or other heart ailment to regain the ability to perform normal functions and activities of life by means of exercise, diet, medication, and a healthy life-style.

Cardiopulmonary arrest: the sudden stoppage of the heartbeat and breathing, causing death within a few minutes unless effective cardiopulmonary resusci-tation is started promptly.

Cardiopulmonary resuscitation: an emergency procedure used to save a person's life when his or her heart and respirations have stopped. The technique involves rhythmic inflation of the lungs alternating with, or accompanied by, simultaneous compressions of the chest over the heart in a specific pattern.

Cardiovascular disease: illness that affects the heart and blood vessels.

Cardiovascular renal disease: kidney disease caused by diseases of the heart and blood vessels.

Cardioversion: the use of electric current to shock the heart into normal rhythm when other methods, such as medication, fail to reverse potentially fatal irregularities of the heart beat.

Carotene: a precursor of vitamin A; serum levels are measured in patients with night blindness and other forms of vit A deficiency.
Normal values: 40-200 µg/dL

Carotid arteriography: an X-ray study of the neck arteries after injection of contrast medium into the carotid artery.

Carpal tunnel syndrome: compression of the median nerve located between the tendons and a ligament of the wrist, causing pain, weakness, and burning or tingling sensations in the hand and fingers.

Carrier: an otherwise healthy person who harbors disease-causing organisms that may be transmitted to others.

Catabolism: the process of breakdown of complex body compounds into simpler ones.

Catalyst: a substance that promotes or speeds up a chemical reaction but is not changed in the process.

Cataract: clouding of the lens in one or both eyes.

Catecholamines: compounds, such as adrenaline and noradrenaline, produced by the medulla (central portion) of the adrenal glands. Catecholamines may be elevated after ingestion of coffee, bananas, and certain drugs, and in patients with pheochromocytoma, a tumor of the adrenal gland.
    Normal values: in urine after 24-hr collection:
        total free catecholamines, 4-126 µg (varies with activity);
        epinephrine, less than 10 µg;
        norepinephrine, less than 100 µg.

Catheterization: a procedure in which a narrow hollow tube is introduced into a body part to examine it; remove fluid or tissue; or introduce fluid, medication, or diagnostic material such as contrast medium.

Catheterization, cardiac: see Cardiac catheterization

Catheterization, urinary: a procedure in which a sterile thin tube (catheter) is passed into the urinary bladder, either to remove urine when the patient cannot urinate normally or to obtain sterile urine for diagnostic tests.

Catheterized urine specimen: a urine specimen used to test for microorganisms in the urinary tract; it is obtained through a catheter under sterile conditions, protected from contamination by organisms elsewhere in or on the patient's body, or on the hands of the person obtaining the specimen.

Cat scratch fever (cat scratch disease): a disease, believed to be caused by a virus, that is transmitted by scratches or bites from apparently healthy cats. Symptoms include swollen lymph nodes, fever, headache, and nausea.

Cauterization: destruction of damaged or superfluous tissue by means of heat, electricity, or a chemical.

CD4 count: a diagnostic procedure done to determine the number of CD4 cells (lymphocytes or T4 helper cells) present in the blood. The test helps to monitor the progress of HIV infection and AIDS: The CD4 cell count decreases as the disease advances.

CD4 percentage: the number of CD4 cells as it relates to a person's total number of lymphocytes (white blood cells). Used to monitor the progress of HIV infection. The percentage of CD4 cells decreases as the disease advances.

Celiac angiography: an X-ray study of the blood vessels of the liver, spleen, stomach, and pancreas after injection of contrast medium.

Celiac disease: a rare intestinal disease that usually develops in small children who are unable to digest the cereal protein gluten.

Cell culture: the process of growing cells in a nutrient solution or material outside the body.

Cellulitis: inflammation of connective tissues.

Celsius (centigrade): a temperature scale on which 0° is the freezing point, and 100° the boiling point, of water.

Central nervous system (CNS): the brain, spinal cord, and nerves that originate from the brain and spinal cord.

Central venous pressure: a test to assess the heart's ability to manage the volume of blood flowing through it. Special equipment is used to measure the trend of central venous pressure, more important in patients who require this measurement than a particular pressure reading by itself.

Cephalin-cholesterol flocculation test: a test for liver disease, based on the reaction between a mixture of the patient's serum and an emulsion of cephalin and cholesterol.
Normal values:
    after 24 hours, negative to 1+;
    after 48 hours, 2+ or less.

Cercarienhullenreaktion: a test done to diagnose and follow-up the parasitic disease schistosomiasis.

Cerebral angiography: an X-ray study of cerebral blood vessels after injection of contrast medium.

Cerebral embolism: sudden blockage of an artery in the brain by material circulating in the bloodstream, such as a blood clot, air, fat, a tumor, or clumps of bacteria. The resulting decrease in blood flow through the artery may lead to a stroke and possibly to death.

Cerebral palsy: a brain defect, usually apparent at birth, that causes varying degrees of difficulty in muscle function and control.

Cerebral thrombosis: the formation or presence of blood clots in an artery inside the brain, which may cause a stroke by cutting off the blood supply to part of the brain.

Cerebrospinal fluid (CSF): the fluid that bathes the brain and spinal canal. It may be examined for the presence of blood, infection, and other abnormalities.

Cerebrospinal fluid cell count: a test to detect infection in the brain or spinal canal.
Normal values: 0-8 cells/μL

Cerebrospinal fluid culture: an incubation in the laboratory of a sample of CSF to determine whether it contains disease-causing microorganisms.

Cerebrospinal fluid scan: a scan of the brain after injection of a radioactive substance into the spinal canal; done to detect spinal fluid leak or abnormalities of the skull.

Cerebrovascular accident (CVA): damage to the brain resulting from blockage or rupture of a cerebral artery, also called a stroke. A CVA may cause loss of consciousness, paralysis, or death, depending on its severity and location and the patient's state of health.

Ceruloplasmin: a protein with which most of the blood's copper is combined. Elevated levels may occur in liver disease, leukemia, and heart attack; decreased levels occur in other forms of liver disease and in nutritional deficiencies.
Normal values: in serum, 23-50 mg/dL.

Cerumen: ear wax.

Cervical intraepithelial neoplasia: a precancerous change of certain cells in a woman's cervix.

Cervical punch biopsy: removal of small amounts of tissue from the cervix (mouth of womb) and uterus (womb) for examination. Abnormal tissue may indicate several types of cancer or other conditions such as inflammation or infection.

Cervicitis: inflammation owing to infection or injury of the cervix, the narrow part (neck) at the lower end of the womb.

Chancroid: a sexually transmitted disease caused by the bacterium *Haemophilus ducreyi*, which produces a small, soft, painful lesion in the genital area.

Chest X-ray: an X-ray done to detect lung disease or to determine the size and position of the heart, ribs, or other internal structures of the chest.

Chickenpox: a highly contagious viral disease, also called varicella, that usually occurs in childhood but may infect adults who did not acquire immunity by having the disease as children. Chickenpox causes eruptions of pustules all over the body and lasts about two weeks.

Chinese restaurant syndrome: a set of symptoms that may occur in people who are sensitive to a spice called monosodium glutamate, often used in Chinese food. Symptoms may include burning sensations in various parts of the body, chest pain, and sometimes a feeling of facial pressure.

***Chlamydia trachomatis*:** an organism that causes a variety of diseases affecting the mucous membranes of the eye and urogenital area. It is transmitted by sexual contact or by direct contact during childbirth or child care.

Chloride: a salt. In blood, it is measured to provide diagnostic information on acid-base balance, osmotic status, and water balance. In CSF, it is measured to detect brain or spinal infection or other abnormalities. In sweat, it is measured to aid in the diagnosis of fibrocystic disease (in which it is elevated). In urine, it is measured to diagnose drug toxicity, dehydration, and some forms of kidney disease (it is decreased with excessive excretion of urine, sweating, diarrhea, or vomiting).
  Normal values:
    in serum, 96-106 mEq/L;
    in CSF,
        adults, 118-132 mEq/L;
        children, 120-128 mEq/L;
    in sweat, 0-30 mmol/L;
    in urine after 24-hr collection, adults, 110-250 mmol/L;

Cholangiography: an X-ray study of the gallbladder and ducts often done in the course of surgery of the gallbladder and related structures.

Cholangitis: inflammation of the bile ducts, the structures that carry bile from its origin in the liver to the gallbladder and the small intestine.

Cholecystitis: inflammation of the gallbladder.

Cholecystography: *oral:* radiographic examination of the gallbladder done after the patient eats a prepared fatty meal and swallows a contrast agent (usually pills) that outlines the gallbladder and nearby structures. *Intravenous:* an X-ray examination of the gallbladder done after injection of radiopaque dye to determine the presence of gallstones.

Choledocholithiasis: the presence of calculi in the common bile duct.

Cholelithiasis: the presence of gallstones in the gallbladder or bile ducts.

Cholera: a serious bacterial disease caused by the organism *Vibrio cholerae* that tends to occur in epidemic form, primarily in Asian countries. It affects the gastrointestinal tract, causing severe, watery diarrhea and massive loss of fluids and electrolytes. A state of collapse results if fluid loss is not promptly replaced.

Cholesterol: a lipid (fatty) substance found in animal tissues and body fluids, important in various metabolic processes, and implicated as a causative factor in arteriosclerosis.

Cholesterol, total: a substance that aids in fat digestion and production of several body hormones. This substance is elevated in certain liver, thyroid, kidney, and other diseases; decreased in certain anemias, glandular deficiencies, and other forms of liver disease. Measurement of the serum level of cholesterol is used primarily to assess the risk of coronary artery disease. (see Lipoproteins for other fatty blood components.) *Normal values:* 150-200 mg/dL, depending on diet and age.

Cholinesterase: a catalytic enzyme that hydrolyzes acetylcholine into choline and acetic acid; it is needed for transmission of nerve impulses of the parasympathetic nervous system. Decreased levels may indicate organic phosphate poisoning, cancer, and liver and certain skin conditions.

Normal values:
in serum, 0.5-1.3 pH units;
in erythrocytes (red blood cells), 0.5-1.0 pH units.

Chorionic villus sampling: a diagnostic method sometimes done 8-10 weeks after the start of pregnancy to discover fetal abnormalities. A catheter (small tube) is inserted through the vagina, cervix, and uterus. Using ultrasound guidance, a small sample of villi (small projections of the sac that surrounds the fetus) is then removed and examined.

Chromatin: the part of a cell's nucleus that can be stained.

Chromatography: a chemical analysis technique in which substances such as hormones, drugs, or enzymes are first separated and then identified by passing them through an adsorbent.

Chromogenic: capable of producing color.

Chromosome: a thread-like body in the nucleus of a living cell that transmits hereditary characteristics.

Chromosome analysis: a test done on white blood cells, bone marrow, or skin cells that have been prepared and chemically treated, for detection of sex identity and various genetic diseases, such as Down syndrome, in the fetus, child, or adult.

Chronic fatigue syndrome: a condition that begins with flu-like symptoms that persist indefinitely. Symptoms may include mild fever, muscle and joint aches, mood swings and inability to function at reduced activity level. The cause is unknown. Treatment consists of rest and relief of symptoms.

Chronic interstitial nephritis: inflammation of the kidneys.

Chronic myelogenous leukemia: a cancerous disease of the white blood cells called myeloblasts.

Chronic obstructive airway disease: long-standing disease of the lungs and respiratory tract, such as emphysema; hinders breathing.

Chronic obstructive pulmonary disease: see Chronic obstructive airway disease.

Chronic persistent hepatitis: inflammation of the liver that persists over long periods of time.

Chronic renal failure: a progressive condition in which the kidneys lose their ability to filter waste from the bloodstream. Alternate means of removing these wastes, such as hemodialysis, peritoneal dialysis, or kidney transplant, must be found in order for the affected person to survive.

Chronic renal insufficiency: a form of kidney dysfunction in which certain waste products are not properly excreted by the body. If this condition persists, accumulation of waste products in the blood will upset fluid and electrolyte balance and lead to symptoms such as fatigue, weakness, and decreased mental alertness.

Chronic respiratory failure: long-term inability of the lungs to function normally, caused by a variety of diseases.

Cineradiography: a process in which fluoroscopic images of moving body parts are projected on an image intensifier, then photographed on a videotape for viewing on a television screen.

Citrate agar hemoglobin electrophoresis: a procedure that separates and identifies various forms of hemoglobin, such as HbA or HbF. HbF is the primary hemoglobin type found in newborns. A high concentration of HbF in adults may indicate early

hereditary anemia. Presence of HbS indicates sickle cell anemia.
Normal adult values:
in venous blood,
HbA, 97-98% of total hemoglobin;
HbA$_2$, 1.5-3.5% of total hemoglobin;
HbF, less than 2% of total hemoglobin;
HbS, none.

Citric acid: a compound similar to ascorbic acid (vitamin C).
Normal values: in serum or plasma, 1.7-3.0 mg/dL.

Clone: the reproduction of a cell in its exact image.

Clostridial gas gangrene: a condition in which wound infection by *Clostridium* bacteria leads to the production of gas and toxins that destroy tissue.

Clotting time: see Bleeding and clotting time.

Coagulase: an enzyme that speeds the clotting process in blood.

Coagulase test: a test done on *Staphylococcus* organisms to determine whether they are producing coagulase.

Coagulation: the process of clotting or clumping of blood.

Coagulation tests: tests performed on whole blood, plasma, or serum to determine the blood's capacity to clot. Abnormal results indicate coagulation defects owing to disease or medication.
Normal values:
bleeding time, 3-10 min (depending on method used);
clot retraction, half the original mass in 2 hr;
dilute blood clot lysis time, 6-10 hr at 37°C;
venous clotting time, 3 tubes, 5-15 min;
whole blood clot lysis time, none in 24 hr;

prothrombin time (PT), 12-14 sec;
partial thromboplastin time (PTT), 60-85 sec (after addition
of PT reagent and ionized calcium.

Coccidioidomycosis: an infection caused by the organism
Coccidioides immitis that may be seen as disseminated (spread
throughout the body) disease in AIDS patients.

Coccidioidomycosis antibodies: antibodies that are found in the
blood of patients with coccidioidomycosis, a fungus infection that
affects the respiratory tract and occasionally other parts of the body
such as skin, bone, and central nervous system.

Coccus: a type of bacterial cell.

Cofactor: a substance that is essential to the function of an
enzyme.

Cold agglutinins: agglutinins that act only at low temperatures;
present in the blood of patients with atypical pneumonia. Using the
agglutination process, a distinction may be made between
Mycoplasma and virus pneumonia.
  Normal value: in serum, a titer of less than 1 : 32.

Cold stimulation test: a test done to diagnose Raynaud's disease,
a circulatory disease of the fingers and, sometimes, the toes, found
more frequently in people who smoke.
  Normal value: finger temperature becomes normal within 15
  min after fingers are removed from an ice solution.

Coliform bacteria: bacteria, such as *Escherichia coli*, that live in
the intestine.

Coliform bacteria infection: an infection with bacteria that normally inhibit the colon (large intestine), especially *Escherichia coli* and members of the *Enterobacter-Klebsiella* group. It may be secondary to infection elsewhere in the body or may be transmitted by transfusion of contaminated blood.

Colonoscopy: an examination of the colon done by inserting a flexible instrument called a fiberoptic endoscope to visualize abnormalities along the entire length of the colon, take tissue samples for diagnosis, or remove small growths.

Colony: a large group of microorganisms grown in a culture medium from a small sample; used for diagnostic purposes or for making vaccines and other preparations for research, treatment, or prevention of disease.

Color vision test: a test done to measure a person's ability to perceive and correctly identify different colors.

Colposcopy: an examination of the vagina and cervix with an endoscope to detect signs of disease.

Coma: a deep unconscious state in which a person is unable to respond to stimuli such as another person's voice or pain. It may result from trauma, illness, poisoning, or an overdose of drugs or alcohol.

Combined fatty acids test: a test done on feces to determine the patient's ability to digest fats.
Normal values: 5-15% of dry matter.

Communicable disease: a disease that can be transmitted from one person to another through direct contact, air vectors, food, body fluids, or excreta.

Complement: a blood protein capable of killing bacteria and other cells or organisms in the presence of an antigen-antibody complex.

Complement assays: a test done on blood to detect deficiencies in the immune system. Increased complement findings may indicate a number of diseases, including rheumatoid arthritis, ulcerative colitis, and diabetes mellitus. Decreased complement findings may indicate such diseases as acute serum sickness, systemic lupus erythematosus, multiple myeloma, and others.
Normal values:
total hemolytic complement, 75-160 U/mL;
C^1 esterase, serum, 2.5-3.8 mg/dL;
C^3, serum, 80-155 mg/dL;
C^4, serum, 13-37 mg/dL.

Complement fixation: the binding of complement by an antigen-antibody complex. This reaction is the basis of diagnostic tests for virus infection, fungus caused lung infection, and a number of other infectious diseases.

Complete blood count (CBC): a blood test done to determine the number of red and white blood cells, and the concentration (hematocrit) and quality of the red cells in a sample of blood.
Normal values in whole blood:
hematocrit,
in men, 40-54%;
in women, 38-47%;
hemoglobin,
in men, 13.5-18.0 g/dL;
in women, 12.0-16.0 g/dL;
red cell count,
in men, 4.6-6.2 million/mm^3;
in women, 4.2-5.4 million/mm^3;
white cell count, 4,500-11,000/mm^3.

Complete bundle branch block: cessation of the electrical impulses governing the heartbeat that normally travel from the heart's upper chambers (auricles) to the lower chambers (ventricles).

Complete heart block: complete lack of transmission of the heartbeat from the auricles to the ventricles.

Compound F: see Cortisol.

Computerized axial tomography (CAT): a radiologic technique in which a radioactive isotope is injected and the radioactive emissions are picked up by the scanning apparatus and transmitted to a computer. An image of the scanned body part is then reconstructed on the screen of a video display terminal.

Computerized electroneuro-ophthalmography: a radiologic technique in which a computerized device is used to generate and control stimuli and patient responses, allowing the diagnosis of such nervous diseases as multiple sclerosis.

Concentration test: a test of the kidney's capacity to concentrate and dilute urine.
Normal values:
>in random urine specimen after fluid restriction,
>>specific gravity, more than 1.025;
>>osmolality, more than 850 mOsm/L.

Condylomata acuminata: a sexually transmitted disease caused by the papilloma virus; also termed genital warts. The warts occur in moist areas, such as inside or outside the penis, inside or outside the female genital organs, the rectum, or the perianal area.

Congenital head disease (CHD): a disease present at birth caused by a defect or malfunction of the heart or adjacent structures.

Congestive cardiac failure: impaired heart function causing retention of fluid in the body; swelling of the legs and feet; shortness of breath; poor circulation of the blood, and other problems.

Congestive heart failure (CHF): a condition caused by the heart's inability to pump blood in the quantities required by the body. Abnormal fluid accumulation occurs in the lungs and other major organs as blood backs up instead of circulating normally.

Conization: removal of a conical piece of tissue.

Constipation: an inability to move the bowels easily. It may be caused by dehydration, insufficient fiber in the diet, poor elimination habits, or gastrointestinal or other illness.

Continuous cycling peritoneal dialysis: an ongoing process in which waste substances are removed from the body of a person with non-functioning kidneys, using the peritoneum (membrane that covers the abdominal cavity) to transfer solution into, and water and soluble waste material out of, the body.

Contraction stress test: see Breast stimulation stress test.

Contrast medium: a liquid or semisolid substance that is radiopaque (meaning it will not allow the passage of X-rays through it); used to make internal structures visible during radiologic examination and on X-ray film.

Convalescent carrier: a person or animal recovering from an infection but still harboring disease-causing microorganisms and capable of transmitting them to others.

Convalescent serum: the serum of a person who has recovered from an infection. It may be given to another person as a preventive measure.

Convulsion: involuntary contraction of the voluntary muscles, also called a seizure. Convulsions may affect the entire body or only a part, such as an extremity. The many possible causes include head injury, high fever, drug or alcohol overdose, and disease.

Coombs' test: a test to detect, and differentiate between, various types of anemias; most commonly used to detect blood incompatibility reactions in pregnant women and their babies.
Normal values:
>direct (in cord blood), no antibodies coating the red blood cells (no complete agglutination);
>indirect (in maternal serum), no antibodies to red blood cell antigens.

Copper: a mineral in blood essential for hemoglobin synthesis; and excreted in urine in increased amounts in certain liver diseases, infections, heart attack, and leukemia and in decreased amounts in Wilson's disease and sprue.
Normal values:
>in serum or plasma,
>>in men, 70-140 µg/dL;
>>in women, 85-155 µg/dL;
>in urine after 24-hr collection, 0-50 µg.

Coproantibodies: antibodies produced in the intestinal tract.

Coproporphyrin: a substance normally excreted in urine in minute amounts; excretion is elevated in liver and certain metabolic diseases.
Normal values:
>in random urine, in adults, 3-20 µg/10 mL;
>in urine after 24-hr collection,
>>in adults, 50-250 µg;
>>in children, 0-80 µg.

Coprozoic: relating to coprozoa, protozoa found in feces.

Coronary arteriography: an X-ray study of the coronary arteries after injection of contrast medium through a catheter.

Coronary artery disease: illness, most often due to arteriosclerosis, that damages the arteries of the heart, reducing the blood flow to areas of the heart muscle (myocardium).

Cor pulmonale: enlargement of the right lower chamber of the heart (ventricle) caused by inadequate lung function; may lead to right-heart failure.

Corticotropin (ACTH) response test: a test in which ACTH is administered (following determination of the baseline cortisol level) to assess the response of the adrenal glands. A failure of cortisol to rise indicates Addison's disease, while an increase above normal indicates Cushing's disease.
 Normal values: an increase above baseline cortisol (5 µg/dL) of more than 7 µg/dL, with a peak level more than 18 µg/dL at 30 min.

Cortisol: also called compound F or hydrocortisone, a principal secretion of the cortex (outer layer) of the adrenal gland; blood or urine levels are measured to detect Addison's disease, adrenogenital syndrome, Cushing's syndrome, and other conditions.
 Normal values:
  in plasma,
   a.m., 5-25 µg/dL;
   p.m., 2-18 µg/dL;
  in urine, 10-100 µg/24 hr.

Coryza: an acute inflammation of the mucous membranes of the nose accompanied by profuse discharge.

Counterstain: a second stain applied over a first for greater staining effect.

C-peptide test: a test done on diabetic patients to determine whether they are able to make their own insulin.
 Normal value: in blood, C-peptide is present.

C-reactive protein: a protein found in the blood of patients with inflammatory diseases; its presence can help determine the cause of rheumatoid arthritis and certain types of pneumonias or other upper respiratory infections.
Normal value: in serum, negative.

Creatine: a compound normally stored in muscle tissue as phosphocreatine; found in small quantities in urine and in larger quantities in children and pregnant women.
Normal values: in urine after 24-hr collection,
in men, 0-40 mg;
in women, 0-100 mg (higher in children and pregnant women).

Creatine phosphokinase: an enzyme present in the heart and skeletal muscles. Blood levels are elevated following a heart attack and in patients with muscular dystrophy and other muscle conditions.
Normal values: in serum,
in men, 55-170 U/L at 37oC;
in women, 30-135 U/L at 37oC.

Creatinine: a protein waste-product elevated in disturbances of kidney function.
Normal values: in urine after 24-hour collection,
in men, 20-26 mg/kg of body weight;
in women, 14-22 mg/kg of body weight.

Creatinine clearance, endogenous: the rate at which the kidneys remove creatinine from the blood, tested to evaluate kidney function.
Normal values: in urine, 115 ± 20 mL/min.

Crossmatching: determining the compatibility of a donor's blood with a recipient's blood prior to blood transfusion.
Normal value: no sign of agglutination (clumping) or hemolysis (destruction) of red blood cells

Cryobiology: the science of biologic effects of very low temperatures.

Cryoglobulins: immunoglobulins that precipitate only in cold temperatures; found mainly in the presence of blood vessel illness. *Normal values:* in serum, negative.

Cryosurgery: a surgical process using a very cold (refrigerated) probe to remove or destroy tissue.

Cryptococcosis: an infection caused by the organism *Cryptococcus neoformans*, usually present in patients whose immune system is depressed, such as those with AIDS.

Cryptosporidiosis: an infection caused by the organism *Cryptosporidium*, which causes an opportunistic infection most often seen in immunocompromised patients such as those with AIDS.

Culdoscopy: a procedure in which an endoscope is passed through the posterior vaginal wall to permit visualization of the female pelvic structures.

Culture: the incubation of a sample of body fluid in a nutrient broth in order to identify microorganisms.

Culture medium: a nourishing substance used to grow microorganisms in the laboratory.

Current procedural terminology (CPT): a set of codes established for every diagnostic test and procedure. Using these codes makes it easier to track costs and patient records for insurance companies, Medicare, doctors and hospitals.

Cushing's syndrome: condition caused by excessive cortisol and other adrenal hormones. Symptoms include a distinctive type of obesity, high blood pressure, muscle wasting and weakness, fragile skin, brittle bones, glucose intolerance, and emotional disorders.

Cyanosis: a bluish appearance of the skin caused by poor circulation, which prevents sufficient oxygen from reaching the tissues.

Cyclic adenosine monophosphate: a cyclic nucleotide; it is measured in urine to check the level of urine enzymes that may indicate an abnormal response to parathyroid hormone.
Normal values: an elevation (3.6-4.0 micro-moles) can indicate a normal response or the presence of hypoparathyroidism; abnormal findings may indicate pseudo-hypoparathyroidism.

Cysteine and cystine: amino acids (protein components); they are elevated in certain metabolic disturbances that can produce kidney and other diseases.
Normal values: in urine after 24-hr collection, 10-100 mg.

Cystic fibrosis: a hereditary disease of children and young adults characterized by abnormal function of the sweat and mucus-secreting glands. It primarily affects the lungs and digestive systems, especially the pancreas.

Cystine, quantitative: a urine test for cystine, rarely found except in patients with certain forms of congenital disease.
Normal value: negative.

Cystitis: inflammation of the urinary bladder.

Cystometrogram: the recording of an x-ray of the urinary bladder for diagnostic purposes.

Cystometrography: measurement of pressure changes inside the urinary bladder with volume over time.

Cystometry: measurement of the urinary bladder's muscular strength.

Cystoscopy: direct visual exam of bladder and part of the urinary tract with a cystoscope, for diagnostic and treatment purposes.

Cystourethrography: a test done with special equipment under sterile (surgical) conditions to investigate disorders of the urinary tract. A thin, lighted tube called a cystoscope is passed through the urethra and into the bladder. Telescopic lenses allow inspection of the internal urethral and bladder tissues. A local anesthetic is given before the start of the procedure. Such conditions as stones in the bladder, polyps, tumors, an enlarged prostate, and strictures of the urethra may be diagnosed.

Cytogenetics: the science of chromosomes and genes.

Cytology: the science of cells.

Cytolysin: a substance able to dissolve living cells.

Cytomegalovirus (CMV) infection: This infection caused by cytomegalovirus may cause such symptoms as enlarged lymph nodes, weakness, fever, and enlarged liver and spleen. In AIDS patients, cytomegalovirus may cause encephalitis, retinitis, diarrhea and weight loss.

Cytoplasm: the portion of a living cell that surrounds the nucleus.

D

Darkfield examination: a test to diagnose syphilis during the first (primary) stage of the disease.
Normal value: in fluid from the lesion, negative for *Treponema* organisms.

Decubitus ulcer: an inflamed sore often found on the skin of elderly, debilitated, bedridden persons with poor circulation. Also known as bedsores or pressure sores, these ulcers occur most frequently in areas subject to pressure, such as the spine, hip, heel, elbow, and buttocks.

Defibrillate (defibrillator): a process (machine) that is used to restart the heartbeat in situations where the heart has stopped due to trauma, illness, or other causes.

Defibrillation: the use of electric current to shock the heart into regular rhythm when it is in fibrillation (a potentially fatal abnormal rhythm) or has stopped beating.

Dehydroepiandrosterone: a sex hormone secreted by the testes and adrenal glands that stimulates development of secondary sex characteristics.
Normal values:
in urine after 24-hr collection,
in men, 0.2-2.0 mg;
in women, 0.2-1.8 mg.

Delirium tremens: a state of alcohol poisoning, brought on by prolonged drinking. Symptoms include trembling; hearing of voices (hallucinations); feelings of being persecuted (paranoia); and exhaustion.

Delta-aminolevulinic acid: see β-aminolevulinic acid.

Dementia: a progressive decline in intellectual function that makes normal thought and activity increasingly difficult.

Dengue: a viral infection usually seen in the tropics and occasionally in southern areas of the United States. Symptoms include chills, high fever, headache, joint and muscle pains, and a rash.

Deoxyribonucleic acid (DNA): a nucleic acid that is an essential component of a chromosome; that carries the genetic information of the organism.

Dexamethasone suppression test: a test performed by giving dexamethasone, then taking blood samples to differentiate between cancer and other types of growths on the adrenal glands. The test can sometimes also determine the presence of mental depression.

Dextrostix: commercially prepared materials used by a diabetic to test his or her blood sugar level.

Diabetes insipidus (pituitary): a disease marked by excessive, dilute urine output and severe thirst, caused by an abnormality of the pituitary gland, one of whose functions is body fluid regulation. Pituitary extract, a synthetic pituitary-like substance, or drugs can be used to treat the disease.

Diabetes mellitus: a metabolic disease in which the body cannot produce or properly utilize insulin, which regulates carbohydrate metabolism. Diabetes is classified into two major types: Type 1, or insulin-dependent diabetes mellitus (IDDM); and Type 2, or non-insulin-dependent diabetes mellitus (NIDDM).

Diabetic ketoacidosis: a complication of diabetes in which free fatty acids in the liver are broken down into substances harmful to the body. Ketoacidosis may lead to decreased blood volume, sweating, nausea, vomiting, mental changes, coma, and death if not treated promptly.

Diacetic acid: a ketone body produced in certain metabolic diseases such as uncontrolled diabetes; also known as acetoacetic acid. *Normal value:* in urine, negative.

Diagnex Blue tubeless gastric analysis: a test done on urine to determine gastric acid secretion. Normal value: some free acid present

Diagnosis: the process of determining a patient's condition or illness. This is done by taking a patient's physical and family history, and conducting a physical examination. Laboratory tests or procedures may also be done to aid the diagnostic process.

Dialysis, hemodialysis: a process involving special equipment that removes waste products from the blood in persons with nonfunctioning kidneys.

Diaphragmatic hernia: a rupture in the dome-shaped partition that divides the chest from the abdomen. It may be treated with medication or surgery.

Diastole: the period during which the heart is at rest, and its chambers fill with blood.

Dick test: a skin test to detect susceptibility to scarlet fever.
Normal values: in skin injected with scarlet fever toxin: negative (no skin reaction; not susceptible).

Differential blood count: a measurement of the percentages of the various types of leukocytes (white blood cells) in a sample of whole blood.
Normal values:
neutrophils, 65% total (58% mature and 7% young);
lymphocytes, 27%;
monocytes, 5%;
eosinophils, 2%;
basophils, 1%.

Differential stain: a stain that allows distinction between various groups of microorganisms.

Digital subtraction angiography: a test using computerized images of blood vessels that lead to the brain and head to determine the adequacy of blood flow (circulation) to the brain.

Digital subtraction echocardiography: an x-ray procedure using computerized techniques and ultra-sound to diagnose various heart problems.

Dilation and curettage (D&C): an operative procedure in which the cervix is dilated and a curette is passed into the uterus for the purpose of obtaining tissue specimens to diagnose a benign or malignant tumor or disease, to remove the products of conception, or for other purposes.

Dinitrochlorbenzene test: a skin test done to determine immune responses. Abnormal reactions (little or no reactions) may indicate deficient immune responses.
   Normal values: normal primary and secondary (delayed) immune responses.

Diodrast clearance: the rate at which the kidneys remove Diodrast, an injected test substance, from the blood or at which the kidneys excrete Diodrast into the urine; it is measured to evaluate kidney function.
   Normal values:
      in serum, 600-720 mL/min;
      in timed urine, 600-720 mL/min.

Diphtheria: a highly contagious bacterial infection of the upper respiratory tract that can prove fatal unless promptly treated with antitoxin and antibiotics. Immunization prevents the disease.

Diplococci: a type of cocci (bacteria) found in pairs.

Direct fluorescent antibody staining for Treponema pallidum: a specific test for syphilis.

Discogram: a radiographic record of an intervertebral disc (a round piece of cartilage separating spinal vertebrae) done to diagnose such conditions as herniation.

Disinfectant: an agent that destroys disease-causing organisms and their products.

Disinfection: the use of a disinfectant to destroy disease-causing organisms and their products.

Disk diffusion test: a test done on blood to determine the susceptibility of a patient's infectious organisms to an anti-infective drug. See Minimal inhibitory concentration.

Disseminated intravascular coagulation (DIC): a process inside blood vessels that sometimes follows certain types of surgery, which produces depletion of substances essential in blood clotting, resulting in profuse bleeding episodes.

Dithionite test: a test done on whole blood to determine the presence of sickle cells.

Diverticulitis: inflammation of the diverticula, abnormal small pouches that sometimes form in the wall of the colon (large intestine). The condition may cause abdominal pain.

Diverticulosis: a condition in which small pouches form in the lining of the colon wall. They may fill with feces and other waste material and become inflamed or infected.

Dead on arrival (DOA): a term used for persons found to be dead at home, in a public place, or who died before reaching the hospital.

Doppler: a technique that uses images made by soundwaves to determine abnormal conditions in tissues, such as obstructions and others.

Doppler ultrasonic flowmeter: device that measures blood flow in blood vessels to diagnose the extent of various circulatory diseases and disorders.

Doppler ultrasonography: a test done to diagnose obstructions and other abnormalities of the heart, arteries, and veins. It also serves to monitor patients who have had arterial or venous surgery such as a bypass.

Down syndrome: a genetic defect that causes characteristic (mongoloid) facial features as well as varying degrees of mental retardation and other defects.

Droplet infection: an infection acquired through the sneezing and coughing of another person.

Drug therapeutic monitoring: tests performed on blood to determine therapeutic levels or identify toxic amounts in blood of drugs such as antibiotics.

Dysfunction: abnormal or impaired function.

Dysfunctional uterine bleeding: bleeding from the womb at times other than menstruation that may be caused by a hormonal or other abnormality or illness.

Dyskinesia: abnormal or difficult voluntary move-ment of muscles, joints or other body parts. May occur as a result of certain medications or illnesses.

Dysmenorrhea: discomfort or pain during menstruation.

Dyspareunia: discomfort or pain during sexual intercourse.

Dyspnea: difficulty in breathing.

E

Echocardiogram: a scan of the heart using ultrasound to record the structure, position, and motion of the heart.

Echoencephalogram: a brain scan using ultrasound to detect such abnormalities as a tumor, clot, or hemorrhage.

Eclampsia: coma and/or seizures that may occur during the last three months of pregnancy or just after giving birth. Symptoms leading to these complications include swelling of tissues caused by fluid retention, high blood pressure, and albumin in the urine.

Ectopic pregnancy: development of the fetus outside the uterus, usually in one of the fallopian tubes.

Eczema: a red, itchy rash that may develop into scales and crusts. Eczema may occur at any age and is often caused by allergies to foods or other substances.

Edema: excessive accumulation of fluid in body tissues accompanied by swelling.

Ejection fraction: the ratio of the amount of blood pumped by the ventricles during one heartbeat to the volume of blood present at the end of the resting phase (diastole).

Elective abortion: the decision by a pregnant woman to have the embryo or fetus removed by one of several different methods that may involve medication, a suction process, or surgery.

Electroanalytic chemistry: a technique that utilizes the interaction of electricity with liquid to measure dissolved substances such as sodium, calcium, and potassium.

Electrocardiogram (ECG): a record of the heart's electrical activity and impulses via monitoring equipment and a printout; important in diagnosing abnormal heart rhythms.

Electrocardiography: see Echocardiogram, Electrocardiogram.

Electroconvulsive therapy: a treatment in which electrical shocks are given to a person with a mental disease such as depression, who has not responded to medication or psychotherapy.

Electroencephalogram (EEG): a record of the brain's electric impulses and activity via monitoring equipment and a printout; important in studying epilepsy and other neurologic conditions.

Electroencephalography: see Electroencephalogram.

Electrolyte: a chemical compound that, when dissolved or melted, breaks up into charged particles (ions) capable of conducting electricity. Electrolytes remain in balance in tissues and body fluids to ensure adequate body functioning. (See Bicarbonate; Calcium; Carbon dioxide; Chloride; Magnesium; Phosphorus; Potassium; and Sodium.)

Electromyogram: a record of electric activity associated with muscle movement; done to evaluate muscle and nerve function and to diagnose dysfunction.

Electromyography: see Electromyogram.

Electrophoresis: a laboratory technique that involves the movement of suspended particles in an electric field; useful for separating and identifying blood substances such as serum proteins, lipoproteins, isoenzymes, and hemoglobin types. See also Citrate agar hemoglobin electrophoresis.

Electrophoresis, protein: a method of determining the presence and quantity of proteins.

Normal values:

in serum,

albumin, 52-65%; 3.2-5.6 g/dL

α_1 globulin, 1.0 : 2.5-5.0%; 0.1-0.4 g/dL

α_2 globulin, 2.0 : 7.0-13.0%; 0.4-1.2 g/dL

β globulin, 8.0-14.0%; 0.5-1.1 g/dL

gamma globulin, 12.0-22.0%; 0.5-1.6 g/dL

in CSF,

prealbumin, 4.1 ± 1.2%

albumin, 62.4 ± 5.6%

α_1 globulin, 1.0 : 5.3 ± 1.2%

α_2 globulin, 2.0 : 8.2 ± 2.0%

β globulin, 12.8 ± 2.0%

gamma globulin, 7.2 ± 1.1%

Electrophysiologic study: a procedure performed to detect electrical impulse disorders of the heart. The process involves placing electrodes into the heart chambers, then stimulating and recording the elec-trical activity in these areas.

Electrophysiology: the study of heart rhythms

Electroshock therapy: see: Electroconvulsive therapy.

Ellsworth-Howard test: a test done by injecting 2 mL of parathyroid extract to determine whether a patient has hypo- or pseudohypoparathyroidism, a glandular condition.

Normal values: in blood, no significant changes after the injection; in urine, no significant changes or, at most, a two-fold increase in urinary phosphorus and AMP secretion in hourly specimens obtained for 3-5 hrs after injection.

Embolism: blockage of blood vessels by a clot or foreign material.

Emergency cardiac compression: a life-saving process used during cardiopulmonary resuscitation to restart a person's heart.

Emergency radiography: X-ray procedures done after a patient has been injured or has developed signs of serious illness, often performed in the emergency department of a hospital.

Emphysema (pulmonary): enlargement of the air sacs in the lungs, causing respiratory difficulty as the condition progresses.

Empyema: the accumulation of pus in a body cavity.

End-stage renal disease: kidney disease that has progressed so that the kidneys no longer remove waste and water from the blood.

Endocardial electric stimulation: a diagnostic procedure providing information about the heart's electric conduction system which is done by placing electrode catheters inside the heart to measure its electric activity.

Endocarditis: inflammation of the lining of the heart, called the endocardium.

Endocrine: ductless; refers to activities and hormonal secretions of ductless glands.

Endogenous: originating in a gland or other internal body part.

Endometritis: inflammation of the mucous membrane that lines the uterus.

Endorectal ultrasound: a procedure in which ultrasound is used to detect a tumor in rectal and nearby areas, such as the prostate.

Endoscopic retrograde biliary drainage: use of a catheter passed into the bile duct to drain bile accumulated there due to illness such as cancer.

Endoscopic retrograde cholangiopancreatography: diagnostic procedure to detect disease of the pancreas, gallbladder, or bile ducts. Performed by passing a small catheter attached to an endoscope into the duodenum and then into the pancreatic duct or common bile duct. Contrast material is injected and X-rays are taken.

Endoscopic variceal sclerotherapy: a treatment done to eliminate varicose veins and prevent bleeding.

Endoscopy: examination of internal body areas (larynx, esophagus, stomach, uterus, rectum, colon) with an endoscope—a device consisting of a tube with a light, refracting mirrors, and other diagnostic and therapeutic accessories—for diagnosis and treatment. See also Fiberoptic endoscopy.

Endotoxin: a toxin liberated during the destruction of bacterial or other microbial cells.

Enteric bacteria: bacteria that live in the gastrointestinal tract.

Enterocolitis: inflammation of the lining (mucous membrane) of the large and small intestines.

Entero test: a diagnostic procedure that checks for abnormalities such as bleeding in the upper gastrointestinal tract. The patient swallows a nylon string encased in a gelatin capsule, which passes down as far as the duodenum. After 3-4 hours, the line is withdrawn and stripped of blood, bile, or other matter, which is then examined; also called a string test.

Enterotoxin: a toxin found in contaminated food that causes vomiting, diarrhea, and possibly serious gastrointestinal illness.

Enteroviruses: viruses that live in the gastrointestinal tract.

Enzyme: a protein secreted by cells that can act as a catalyst, changing or modifying other body secretions and processes without being changed itself.

Enzyme-linked immunosorbent assay (ELISA): a test capable of detecting and measuring levels of hormones, drugs, and various other biologic materials in body fluids. Most often used to monitor blood levels of drugs, but now also used to test for the presence of human immunodeficiency virus (HIV) antibody. If the test is positive for HIV antibodies, a Western blot test is done for confirmation.

Eosinophils: see White blood cell count, differential.

Epidemic: an infection that attacks a large group of people; it typically starts in one local area and then spreads to larger segments of a population, sometimes to other countries or even worldwide.

Epidemiology: the science of tracking widespread contagious and other diseases and conditions.

Epididymitis: inflammation of the structure at the back of the testes that collects sperm from the testicle.

Epidural hemorrhage: bleeding in the cranium outside the dura mater, the tough, fibrous outer coat of the brain.

Epiglottitis: inflammation and swelling of the leaf-shaped piece of fibrous cartilage (epiglottis) that covers the opening of the larynx (voice box) during swallowing to prevent solids or liquids from getting into the trachea.

Epilepsy: a neurologic condition in which abnormal electric activity in the brain triggers seizures of varying severity.

Epinephrine: an adrenal hormone, somewhat elevated in certain psychiatric illnesses, and indicative of pheochromocytoma (a tumor of the adrenal gland) when sharply elevated.
Normal values: in urine, less than 10 μg/24 hr; norepinephrine, less than 100 μg/24 hr.

Epstein-Barr virus: a herpesvirus, also believed to cause mononucleosis.

Erythrocyte: red blood cell.

Erythrocyte Court: a count of erythrocytes (red blood cells) in a sample of whole blood.
Normal values: in men, 4.6-6.2 million/mm^3; in women, 4.2-5.4 million/mm^3

Erythrocyte hemolysis test: a test of the susceptibility of red blood cells to hemolysis; this is an indication of blood levels of vitamin E, which may be deficient in anemias, infertility, and malnutrition.
Normal values: in plasma, 0.5 mg/dL.

Erythrocyte indices: measures of size and hemoglobin concentration of red blood cells.
Normal values:
    mean corpuscular volume: 82-98 cubic microns (fluid)
    mean corpuscular hemoglobin: 27-31 pg
    mean corpuscular hemoglobin concentration: 32-36%

Erythrocyte sedimentation rate (ESR): rate at which erythrocytes settle in unclotted (freshly drawn) whole blood; indicates presence and degree of various inflammatory diseases and infections.
Normal values:
    in men under 50: less than 15 mm/hr
    in men over 50: less than 20 mm/hr
    in women under 50: less than 20 mm/hr
    in women over 50: less than 30 mm/hr

Esophageal acidity: a test that determines the adequacy of the lower esophageal sphincter.
Normal value: pH over 5.

Esophageal manometry (esophageal motility test): a diagnostic test of esophageal function in which pressures are measured at various points inside the esophagus by passing water-filled catheters through the mouth to the stomach to determine abnormal esophageal conditions.

Esophagitis: inflammation of the esophagus, the muscular tube that connects the pharynx (the cavity just behind and below the mouth) to the stomach.

Esophagogastroduodenoscopy: endoscopic examination of the length of the gastrointestinal tract extending from the esophagus to the duodenum.

Esophagoscopy: examination of the esophagus with a scope to detect injury, a growth, or other abnormality.

Esophagram: a diagnostic procedure in which air and barium are introduced into the esophagus and the organ is X-rayed to detect abnormalities.

Estriol: a test done on blood or urine to determine whether a pregnant woman's placenta is functioning adequately.
Normal values:
in blood,
at 30-32 wk, 2-12 ng/mL
at 33-35 wk, 3-19 ng/mL
at 36-38 wk, 5-27 ng/mL
at 39-40 wk, 10-30 ng/mL
in urine,
at 30 wk, at least 9 mg/24 hr; subsequent measurements, plotted on a graph, show a steady increase in levels.

Estrogen receptor test: a test of whether a patient's cancer is stimulated by (responds to) estrogen, performed to determine whether hormonal treatment will be helpful.

Estrogens, fractionated: estrogenic hormones individually measured in urine.
> *Normal values:* in urine after 24-hr collection (nonpregnant, mid-cycle woman):
>> estrone (E1), 4-31 µg
>> estradiol (E2), 0-14 µg
>> estriol (E3), 2-30 µg

Estrogens, total: estrogenic hormones measured together in urine.
> *Normal values:* in urine after 24-hr collection:
>> in men, 4-25 µg
>> in women, ovulation, 25-100 µg
>>> luteal peak, 22-105 µg
>>> menses, 4-25 µg
>>> pregnancy, up to 45,000 µg
>>> postmenopause, 14-20 µg

Ethosuximide: an anticonvulsant medication monitored in plasma to determine steady-state levels (reached 4-7 days after treatment is started).
> *Therapeutic values:* 40-100 µg/mL.

Etiocholanolone: sex hormone secreted by the testes and adrenal glands.
> *Normal values:*
>> in urine after 24-hr collection:
>>> in men, 1.4-5.0 mg
>>> in women, 0.8-4.0 mg

Etiology: cause, usually of a disease.

Evoked potential monitoring: a method of electronically measuring brainwaves and impulses from specific nerve pathways in certain parts of the body. During surgery on the brain or spinal cord, this procedure can prevent inadvertent damage to healthy nervous tissue. Also helps to diagnose neurologic diseases.

Exchange transfusion: the repeated removal of small amounts of blood, followed by substitution of like amounts of blood from a number of donors, until a large portion of the body's blood has been replaced.

Excretory urogram: see Intravenous pyelogram.

Exercise electrocardiography (stress test): a test done to determine the functional capacity of the heart in patients who have no symptoms and to help find the cause of chest pain. This test is also used to set up an appropriate exercise program for people who have a healthy heart, as well as those who have heart disease, to strengthen the heart and at the same time prevent further damage through excessive exercise.

Exercise stress testing: See: Exercise electro-cardiography.

Exophthalmometry: a test done on the eyes to measure whether and to what extent they protrude beyond their normal position. Abnormal protrusion may be caused by infection, thyroid disease, and certain blood disorders.
Normal values: 12-20 mm.

Exotoxin: a poison secreted by disease-causing microorganisms into their environment, such as the host's body.

Extracapsular cataract extraction: removal of the central portion of the capsule (containing the lens of the eye), along with aspiration of the cloudy lens, leaving the posterior portion of the capsule in place. This process allows the placement of an intraocular lens to replace the one that has been removed.

Extracellular: outside the cell.

Extracorporeal irradiation of blood: a process of removing blood from the body, subjecting it to radiation, then returning it to the patient. Done in diseases such as cancer of the lymphatic system.

Extracorporeal shockwave lithotripsy: a treatment method for the removal of urinary or kidney stones. A device called a lithotriptor is used in combination with other equipment to pulverize the stone(s) by means of electrical shock waves, elimi-nating the need for surgical extraction of the stone.

Extractable nuclear antigen antibodies: ribonucleoprotein antibodies; anti-Smith antibodies; Sjögren's antibodies. A test is done on blood to determine the presence of autoimmune disease and to help differentiate between various antibodies found in different autoimmune diseases.

Normal values: negative for ribonucleoprotein antigen (RNP); anti-Smith antigen (anti-SM); and Sjögren's antigen (SS-A,SS-B)

Eye sonogram: a test using ultrasound to detect diseases of the eye.

F

Fahrenheit: temperature scale on which freezing point of water is 32○F and the boiling point of water is 212○F. One degree Fahrenheit (1○F) equals 5/9th of one degree Celsius (centigrade, C).

False negative: a term used to describe an inaccurate negative laboratory test result.

False positive: a term used to describe an inaccurate positive laboratory test result.

Fasting blood sugar: see Glucose, fasting.

Fat embolism: obstruction of an artery by a fat globule released from bone. Symptoms may occur immediately or within 2-3 days after surgery or trauma. Symptoms include increased heart and respiratory rates, fever, shock, and a fine red rash on the upper body.

Fat, neutral (in blood): measurement of fats, such as triglycerides, in the blood, or in feces to check for digestive or pancreatic disturbances.
Normal values:
> in serum or plasma, 0-200 mg/dL
> in 72-hr collection of feces, 1-5% of dry matter

Fat, quantitative: a urine test for fat, present only in patients with kidney abnormalities. *Normal value:* negative

Fat, total: the fat content of the feces; measured to determine whether fat is being absorbed normally and to check for disease states causing abnormal fat levels, such as nontropical sprue or pancreatic disease.
Normal values: in 72-hour collection of feces, 0-25% of weight of specimen; average less than 6 g/24 hrs.

Fatty acids, free: lipid (fatty) derivatives measured in feces to determine a person's ability to digest fats.
Normal values: 5-13% of dry matter

Fatty acids, total: lipid (fatty) derivatives, including saturated and unsaturated fatty acids, measured in serum when disturbances of fat metabolism are suspected.
Normal values: 190-420 mg/dL

Fatty acids, total free: measurements of blood levels of lipid (fatty) fractions stored in adipose tissues.
Normal values:
in serum, 9-15 mmol/L
in plasma, 300-480 µEq/L

Fatty liver: a condition in which fatty droplets accumulate in liver cells, destroying the cells. Fatty liver may accompany alcoholism and a variety of other diseases.

Febrile agglutination: a test done on blood to determine the presence of antibodies to specific organisms that cause infection, and to discover the cause of a fever without a known cause. Performed specifically for the presence of these organisms: *Salmonella, Francisella tularensis, Brucella*, rickettsial virus. A series of tests may be needed to detect a specific infection.
Normal values:
Salmonella antibody, a titer less than 1 : 80
Brucellosis antibody, a titer less than 1 : 80
Tularemia antibody, a titer less than 1 : 40
Rickettsial antibody, a titer less than 1 : 40

Feces: stool, bowel movement, intestinal discharge.

Ferric chloride test: a test done on urine to check for a type of metabolic deficiency called phenylketonuria, which causes mental retardation and poor skin and hair pigmentation.

Normal value: no change in the color of urine when a few drops of a strong acid and 1 mL of 5-10% ferric chloride solution are added to 5 mL of urine.

Ferritin: a blood protein that contains iron; measured to determine the amount of iron stored in the bone marrow, and to diagnose the causes of anemia or unexplained weakness.

Normal values: in serum, 20-270 µg/L.

Fetal alcohol syndrome: various symptoms and conditions affecting the unborn child of an alcoholic mother. After delivery, the baby may be mentally retarded and have multiple physical abnormalities.

Fetal monitoring, external: a test done with external equipment to evaluate how well a fetus is doing in the mother's womb, and to detect early fetal problems. The test measures the unborn baby's heartbeat and the mother's uterine contractions during labor.

Normal values:
range of baby's heartbeat, 120-160 bpm;
contraction stress test, 3 contractions within 10 min without late deceleration.

Fetal monitoring, internal: a test using an internal monitor to determine fetal well-being by measuring fetal heartbeat and the mother's contractions. More definitive than the external fetal monitoring procedure, this test places an electrode through the mother's vagina and dilated cervix into the baby's scalp. A catheter is then filled with fluid and inserted about 1-2 cm into the cervix, next to the baby's head, and connected to an electric measuring device. This allows determination of changes in the fetal heartbeat, in the pressure and frequency of the mother's uterine contractions, and indicates fetal conditions during labor. *Normal values:* fetal heart rate (FHR) 120-160 bpm; 5-25 bpm variability within range.

α₁-Fetoprotein: a protein normally found in appreciable amounts only in the blood of pregnant women, fetuses, and infants. Certain illnesses cause elevated levels in adults. Abnormally increased levels in serum and amniotic fluid during pregnancy may indicate fetal abnormalities.

Normal values: in serum, in adults and children older than 1 yr, less than 40ng/mL.

Fever of unknown origin (FUO): elevated temperature whose cause is not known.

Fiberoptic endoscopy: the use of an endoscope—a flexible tube able to bend light rays—to inspect the interior of a body cavity or organ. Because it bends light rays, the scope can be used to see around corners and other obstacles to diagnose the location and type of disease and to perform operative and other therapeutic procedures. See also Endoscopy.

Fibrillation: rapid, ineffective contractions of the heart, caused by abnormal transmission of electrical impulses from the upper to the lower chambers of the heart. Usually caused by heart disease.

Fibrinogen: a protein involved in the blood clotting process.
Normal values: in plasma, 200-400 mg/dL.

Fibrin split product (FSP) (fibrinogen degradation product): a blood component; a test is done to detect a variety of conditions associated with the blood clotting mechanisms in a number of situations that may involve pregnancy, trauma, heart disease, and others.

Normal values:
in screening assay, less than 10 µg/mL FSP;
in a quantitative assay, less than 3 µg/mL.

Fifth disease: a relatively mild illness, most prevalent in children from four to 12 years old, consisting of a generalized rash, usually with little or no fever; it is believed to be caused by a virus.

Filariasis: a tropical disease caused by the parasitic worm Filaria, whose larvae are carried from one person to another by mosquitoes, mites, or flies. Once inside the human body, the grown worms live in the tissues of the lymphatic system, where they cause swelling, inflammation, and pain. The infection may enormously increase the size of a body part, such as an arm or leg.

Fixation of tissue: the preservation of body tissue in preservative solution in preparation for microscopic or other examination.

Flame photometry: a laboratory technique involving the use of electric particles (cations and anions) and light measurements to measure such substances as sodium, potassium, and lithium.

Fluorescein angiography: a test using a special camera to photograph blood vessels in the eye. These pictures help to diagnose certain eye disorders that may involve inflammation, circulatory problems, or tumors.
> *Normal values:* normal appearance of the interior structures of the eye, normal circulation in the eye's blood vessels, and absence of leakage from any of the retinal blood vessels

Fluorescent eye stain: an eye test to detect injury or other abnormality in the cornea or to aid in fitting contact lenses.
> *Normal value:* no evidence of dye remains after tears have passed over the area.

Fluorescent immunoassay: a laboratory test using fluorescein-labeled antibodies to detect and diagnose various infectious diseases.

Fluorescent treponemal antibody absorption test: a blood test for *Treponema pallidum*, the organism that causes syphilis.
> *Normal value:* in serum, negative.

Fluoride: a fluorine compound excreted in urine if present in the system. *Normal value:* urine after 24-hr collection, less than 1 mg.

Fluorometry: a laboratory technique for measuring substances that become fluorescent in ultraviolet light or when exposed to strong radiant energy. It is used primarily when measuring in very small units such as micrograms or nanograms per milliliter, as occurs in tests for urinary estrogens and catecholamines.

Fluoroscopy: a radiographic technique used to study the functions of internal body structures by projection of images onto a fluorescent screen.

Folate: a folic acid salt. Folate deficiency may occur with alcoholism, taking birth control pills, malnutrition, and certain types of anemia. Deficiency is detected by measuring blood levels by bioassay.
Normal values:
  in serum, 2.2-17.3 ng/mL
  in erythrocytes, 169-707 ng/mL

Folic acid: a vitamin needed to prevent anemias; deficiency may occur with alcoholism, taking birth control pills, malnutrition, and certain diseases. Deficiency is detected by measuring blood levels of folates by bioassay.
Normal values: in serum, 5-25 ng/mL (bioassay).

Follicle-stimulating hormone (FSH): a sex hormone that stimulates the development of egg and sperm cells.
Normal values: in urine after 24-hr collection:
  in women,
    adult, 4-30 mU/mL
    prepubertal, less than 10 mU/mL
    postmenopausal, 40-250 mU/mL
  in men, 4-25 mU/mL

Forced expiratory volume: see Timed forced expiratory volume.

Formiminoglutamic acid: an intermediate product in histidine metabolism; elevated in the urine of patients with deficiency of vitamin B$_{12}$ or folates.
Normal values: less than 3 mg/24 hr after taking 15 grams of 1-histidine, 4 mg/8 hr.

Fragile X syndrome: inherited mental delay caused by a defective gene.

Fragility test: see Osmotic fragility test.

Fructose: a natural sugar excreted in urine.
Normal values: in urine after 24-hr collection, 30-65 mg.

Fulminating infection: a sudden, overwhelming infection.

Fumigation: sterilization of an object or area by exposure to gas fumes.

Funduscopy: examination of the eye with an ophthalmoscope.

Fungal serology: a test done on blood to detect the presence of fungal infections or to monitor the treatment of such infections.
Normal values: a titer, in which no fungal infections are present.

Fungus: a microbe vegetable organism that subsists on molds and other living matter. Some fungi can cause disease.

G

Galactorrhea: excessive discharge of milk from the breast.

Galactose: a milk sugar derivative.
Normal values: in whole blood, in adults, less than 20 mg/dL; none in children.

Gallbladder series: a series of X-ray studies of the gallbladder and related structures; done after the patient swallows contrast medium that outlines the parts to be studied.

Gallium scan: a test done by a nuclear scanning device and a special (gamma scintillation) camera, after an intravenous infusion of a small amount of radioactive gallium is started. The results of the test indicate cancer in various body parts (primary, spreading, or recurrent); infection or inflammation, and liver disorders.
Normal values: no abnormalities visualized.

Gamete intrafallopian transfer: a treatment for infertility. The procedure consists of removing several eggs from the mother, and combining them immediately with a large number of sperm. The mixture is then inserted in the woman's fallopian tube to allow fertilization. If the procedure is successful, the fertilized egg (zygote) proceeds to the uterus where it implants, and develops into an embryo, fetus, and, eventually, a newborn baby.

Gamma globulin: a blood protein fraction that contains antibodies.
Normal values: in serum, 0.5-1.6 g/dL.

Gangrene: the death of body tissues caused by infection, trauma, or other condition resulting in loss of blood supply.

***Gardnerella* (bacterial vaginosis):** a sexually transmitted disease caused by *Gardnerella vaginalis* that may cause a variety of genital symptoms.

Gas chromatography: a laboratory procedure that separates various gases in a two-step process.

Gastric analysis: analysis of fluid aspirated from the stomach to diagnose various diseases or to determine the types and quantities of drugs ingested in an overdose.

Gastric culture: a test done to confirm the presence of tuberculosis. It may also be done to help determine the cause of certain bacterial infections present in a newborn infant's blood.
Normal value: no bacterial or tuberculosis organisms present.

Gastric fluid, basal acid output: a test done to measure the total output of stomach acid in an hour, after the patient has been intubated.
Normal values: 0-6 mEq/hr.

Gastric fluid, basal acid output: maximal acid output ratio: the ratio of basal to maximal acid output; if greater than normal, it may indicate various diseases of the stomach or intestines.
Normal values: less than 0.4

Gastric fluid, fasting residual volume: the residual volume of gastric acid secretion measured after 12 hours of fasting.
Normal values: 20-100 mL

Gastric fluid, maximal acid output: the measurement of stomach acid secretion following stimulation by injection of histamine. If maximal levels are elevated, anemia, stomach infection, or other stomach disease may be present. *Normal values:* 5-40 mEq/hr

Gastric fluid, pH: a measure of the acidity or alkalinity of gastric fluid.

Gastric ulcer: see Ulcer.

Gastrin: a hormone secreted by the pylorus (muscular coat that surrounds the lower outlet of the stomach). This hormone stimulates the production and secretion of hydrochloric acid in the stomach. Elevated levels indicate the presence of a number of disease states. *Normal values:* 40-200 pg/mL

Gastroenteritis: inflammation of the lining of the stomach and intestines.

Gastroesophageal reflux: regurgitation of stomach contents into the food tube (esophagus).

Gastrointestinal hemorrhage: bleeding somewhere in the stomach and/or intestines.

Gastrointestinal series: a series of X-ray studies of the esophagus, stomach, and small bowel; done after the patient swallows barium contrast medium to outline the parts to be studied.

Gastroscopy: an examination of the stomach and upper gastrointestinal tract with a gastroscope.

Generalized infection: an infection that affects the entire body.

Generalized lymphadenopathy: enlargement of lymph nodes throughout the body, which may occur with various infectious diseases such as infectious mononucleosis, cytomegalovirus infection, toxoplas-mosis, and others.

Genetic: carried by the genes; inherited.

Genital warts: see Condylomata acuminata.

Genitourinary: pertaining to the genital and urinary tract or system.

Germ: a microbe that may cause disease.

German measles (rubella): a usually mild infectious viral disease seen mainly in children and young adults. Major symptoms are a red body rash, swollen lymph glands in the neck, and mild fever. The disease is dangerous if contracted by a woman during early pregnancy, since it may cause severe congenital defects in the baby. Vaccination prevents the disease.

Germicide: a substance that kills microbes.

Giardiasis: intestinal infection caused by the parasite *Giardia lamblia*. It often produces no symptoms but may cause diarrhea, flatulence, and abdominal discomfort. Drugs are available to treat the infection.

Giemsa's stain: a solution for staining microorganisms such as protozoa, rickettsiae, and viral inclusion bodies, to make them detectable in laboratory samples.

GI series: see Gastrointestinal series.

Glaucoma: an eye disease that causes elevated pressure inside the eye. If not treated, blindness may result.

Globulins: a group of blood proteins that are soluble in various weak salt solutions but insoluble in water. Each type of globulin has a different biochemical function. See Electrophoresis, protein.

Globulins (in cerebrospinal fluid): measurement of globulin fraction in cerebrospinal fluid.
Normal values: qualitative, negative; quantitative, 6-16 mg/dL.

Globulins, total: measurement of blood levels of the entire group of globulins.
Normal values: in serum, 2.3-3.5 g/dL

Glomerulonephritis: inflammation of the tiny glomeruli (arterial capillaries) of the kidneys, which pass water and dissolved chemicals from blood into the renal tubules for filtration of wastes. The condition interferes with normal kidney function.

Glucagon test: a test done to determine the presence of hypo-glycemia (low blood sugar) due to excessive insulin in the blood, produced either by excessive insulin administration or by a tumor.
Normal values: in blood, 50-100 mg/dL increase in blood glu-cose if patient is given 1 mg of glucagon 6-8 hr after eating; glucose level peaks at 45 min and returns to normal within 2 hr.

Glucose: a natural sugar found in cerebrospinal fluid. CSF levels are measured to detect abnormal conditions of the spinal cord and brain. Levels are decreased in meningitis.
Normal values:
in urine,
quantitative, less than 500 mg/24 hr
qualitative, negative
in CSF, 50-75 mg/dL (20 mg/dL less than serum)

Glucose difference, synovial fluid-blood: see Synovial fluid.

Glucose, fasting: the measurement of blood sugar levels after a 12-hour fast; done to diagnose diabetes.
Normal values:
in serum or plasma, 70-110 mg/dL
in whole blood, 60-100 mg/dL

Glucose oxidase: a urine test done with a chemically treated paper strip that detects the presence of sugar in urine.
Normal value: no glucose found

Glucose-6-phosphate dehydrogenase: a red blood cell enzyme; levels are decreased in a type of anemia.
Normal values:
in erythrocytes (red blood cells),
351 ± 60.6 U/10^{12} RBC or 4.11 ± 0.71 U/mL RBC
in whole blood, 12.1 ± 2.9 U/g Hb

Glucose, qualitative: a urine test for glucose, present in metabolic diseases such as diabetes.
Normal values: negative or trace

Glucose tolerance test (intravenous): a test done to determine one's ability to metabolize glucose. A 25-50% solution of glucose is given intravenously over a period of 15 minutes. The amount infused depends on the patient's weight.
Normal values: in blood, initial glucose level is not elevated; the level does not exceed 250 mg/dL by the end of the infusion, is lower than the initial level at the end of 2 hours, and returns to the pre-infusion value by 3 to 4 hours.

Glucose tolerance test (oral): a metabolic test in which a fasting patient drinks a quantity of glucose. Blood sugar levels are then measured at intervals of 1/2, one, two, three, and four hours.
Normal values:
in urine, negative or trace
in serum or plasma, fasting, 70-110 mg/dL
at 30 min, 30-60 mg/dL above fasting level
at 60 min, 20-50 mg/dL above fasting level
at 120 min, 5-15 mg/dL above fasting level
at 180 min, fasting level or below

γ-glutamyltransferase: an enzyme involved in the transfer of amino acids across the cell membrane; test is done on blood to assess liver function, help in the differential diagnosis between liver and skeletal conditions, and aid in the diagnosis of liver ailments.
Normal values:
in men, 6-32 U/L
in women, 4-18 U/L

γ-glutamyl transpeptidase: see γ-Glutamyltransferase

Glutathione: enzyme; its deficiency may lead to hemolytic anemia.
Normal values: in whole blood, 24-37 mg/dL.

Glycosylated hemoglobin test: measurement of a subgroup of hemoglobin to monitor long-term metabolic control of glucose. The results reflect mean blood glucose concentrations during the preceding several weeks. The test is used primarily to monitor diabetes therapy and compliance with treatment.

Gonadotropins, pituitary: hormones secreted by the pituitary gland that stimulate the ovaries or testes. They include follicle-stimulating hormone (FSH) and luteinizing hormone (LH).
Normal values: in urine after 24-hr collection:
FSH,
in women, 4-30 U/L
postmenopausal, 40-250 U/L
in men, 4-25 U/L
LH,
in women, premenopausal, 5-22 U/L
midcycle, 3 times baseline
postmenopausal, less than 30 U/L
in men, 6-18 U/L

Gonadotropin-releasing hormone: a hormone originating in a region of the brain (hypothalamus) that stimulates production of another hormone (gonadotropin) in the pituitary gland, also located in the brain.

Gonadotropin stimulation test: a test performed to determine the cause of hypogonadism (underdevelopment of the male sex organs). *Normal values:* in plasma 1 day after daily intramuscular (IM) injection of 2,000 IU of chorionic gonadotropin for 4 days, testosterone levels at least double the value before test (300-1,000 mg/dL).

Gonococcal urethritis: an infection of the urethra caused by gonorrhea.

Gonococcus: the organism that causes gonorrhea.

Gonorrhea: a sexually transmitted disease caused by the gonococcus organism. It can be cured relatively quickly during its early stages. It may cause urethral discharge in men, vaginal discharge in women, arthritis-like symptoms, damage to a woman's pelvic organs, and sterility, as well as other symptoms.

Gout: a form of arthritis that most often occurs in men and is caused by excessive amounts of uric acid in the blood. The excess uric acid may be deposited in joint cartilage and other tissues, where it can cause inflammation, swelling, and severe pain.

Gram-negative microorganisms: microorganisms that do not retain the violet dye used in the Gram stain method but instead take the color of the counterstain.

Gram-positive microorganisms: microorganisms that retain the violet dye used in the Gram stain method and do not accept the counterstain.

Gram stain: a staining procedure used in the laboratory to distinguish between different types of microorganisms; see above.

Granuloma inguinale: a sexually transmitted disease (infection) caused by *Calymmatobacterium (Donovania) granulomatis* that may cause a variety of genital or other symptoms.

Growth hormone deficiency: inadequate amounts of the growth hormone, which may stunt a child's normal growing pattern.

Growth hormone suppression test: a test done on blood, after the patient drinks concentrated glucose solution, to assess pituitary human growth hormone (HGH) secretion. Elevated levels may confirm gigantism (excessive growth).
Normal values:
> in adults, negative HGH, 3 ng/mL within 1/2-2 hr;
> in children, rebound stimulation is possible within 2-5 hr.

Grouping, typing: the classification of specific microbes, blood types, cells, or genetic components according to certain common characteristics.

Guiac test: a test performed on feces or urine to detect occult blood in the intestinal or urinary tract. Guiac, a wood resin, is the reagent used in the laboratory procedure.
Normal values:
> in feces after three days of a meat-free diet, negative;
> in urine, negative.

Guanase: an enzyme found in the blood that is sometimes markedly elevated in patients with hepatitis and other types of liver disease and in infectious mononucleosis.
Normal values: in serum, less than 3 nmol/mL/min.

Guthrie bacterial inhibition assay: a blood or urine test for phenylalanine, an amino acid. Elevated levels are seen in patients with phenylketonuria, an inherited enzyme deficiency that causes mental retardation if not diagnosed and treated soon after birth.
Normal values:
> in blood, negative to trace;
> in urine, negative.

Gynecologic: pertaining to the female reproductive system.

H

Hairy cell leukemia: a form of cancer of the white blood cells that are produced by the lymphatic system.

Hairy leukoplakia: whitish spots that may occur in the mouth of HIV-infected persons.

Half-life: the length of time required for a given isotope's radioactivity to decay to half its original strength.

Ham test (acidified serum lysis test): a test done on blood to detect a particular cause of anemia, called paroxysmal nocturnal hemoglobinuria (PNH), in which destroyed red blood cells are found in the urine, generally for several days in a row, more often during the night. This problem occurs irregularly, together with other symptoms such as headache and abdominal and back pain.
Normal value: no destroyed blood cells found

Hansen's disease (leprosy): a chronic, inflammatory, infectious disease primarily found in tropical and subtropical countries but also in the southern United States. The disease is caused by the organism *Mycobacterium leprae,* which produces lesions of the skin, mucous membranes, and peripheral nervous system.

Hapten: a specific portion of an antigen molecule.

Haptoglobin: a blood protein that combines with hemoglobin; a low level indicates a breakdown of red blood cells, which may occur in certain diseases, snakebite, or drug ingestion. Levels are increased in some inflammatory conditions.
Normal values: in serum, 100-200 mg/dL.

HCG radioreceptor assay: a reliable, simple urine test to diagnose early pregnancy, ectopic pregnancy, and missed abortion. Human chorionic gonadotropin (HCG) is found only in pregnancy or in HCG-producing tumors.

Normal values:
> negative within 2 hr if the patient is not pregnant;
> positive within 1 hr if the patient is pregnant.

Head trauma: injury to the skull and brain.

Heart block: a disorder of the electrical system that initiates and regulates the transmission of the heartbeat from the upper chamber of the heart (atrium) to the lower chamber (ventricle).

Heart catheterization: see Cardiac catheterization.

Heart scan: a scan of the heart done after injection of a radioactive substance into a vein, to determine size, shape, and location; to diagnose pericarditis (inflammation and fluid accumulation around the heart); or to view the heart's chambers. A blood pool scan can measure damage sustained after a heart attack.

Heatstroke (sunstroke): a disturbance of the body's heat-regulating mechanism caused by prolonged exposure to high temperatures. Symptoms include high fever, absence of sweating, and collapse, sometimes culminating in convulsions, coma, and death.

Heinz bodies: molecules that damage or destroy red blood cells; they may be the cause of hemolytic anemia, a type of anemia caused by premature destruction of red blood cells.

Normal value: no Heinz bodies found

Hemagglutination inhibition test: a test done on urine to determine the presence or absence of pregnancy.

Normal values: clumping of red blood cells sensitized to HCG (human chorionic gonadotropin) and anti-HCG serum in the urine sample.

Hematocrit: the relative volume of red blood cells in whole blood.
Normal values:
in venous blood,
in men, 40-54%
in women, 38-47%

Hematogenous: originating or carried in the blood.

Hematology: the science of blood, blood-forming organs, and blood diseases.

Hematuria: blood in the urine.

Hemianopsia: defective vision or blindness in one half of the visual field in one or both eyes.

Hemodialysis: see: Dialysis.

Hemoglobin: the oxygen-carrying protein pigment in red blood cells; found in the urine only in the presence of an abnormality or disease of the genitourinary tract, or in hemolytic anemia.
Normal values:
in serum or plasma,
qualitative, negative;
quantitative, 0.5-5.0 mg/dL
in whole blood,
in women, 12.0-16.0 g/dL
in men, 14.0-18.0 g/dL
in urine, negative.

Hemoglobin A$_2$: a type of hemoglobin; it is elevated in various blood diseases.
Normal values: in blood, 1.5-3.5% of total hemoglobin.

Hemoglobin derivatives: a test done on blood to determine whether abnormal hemoglobin constituents are causing a lack of oxygen in body cells. May be needed for individuals who are subject to carbon monoxide exposure. If abnormal hemoglobin constituents are detected, immediate treatment must be given.

Normal value: no abnormalities found.

Hemoglobin F: fetal hemoglobin; in adults or children, abnormally elevated levels may indicate various blood diseases and conditions, including aplastic anemia, leukemia, and thalassemia, a type of hemolytic anemia.

Normal values: in blood, hemoglobin F is the major constituent of fetal blood, but normally constitutes less than 2% of hemoglobin in adults.

Hemoglobin, glycosylated: see: Glycosylated hemoglobin.

Hemogram: a laboratory record, either written or graphic, of the differential blood count, with special emphasis on the size, shape, special characteristics, and numbers of the solid constituents of the blood. See also Complete blood count (CBC).

Hemolysis: the dissolving or destruction of red blood cells by a chemical substance or disease.

Hemophilia: a hereditary illness in which the blood does not clot, or does so very slowly, predisposing the victim to spontaneous bleeding or prolonged bleeding following trauma or surgery.

***Haemophilus influenzae* infection:** illness caused by the *Haemophilus influenzae* organism, including some respiratory infections, ear infections, and infection of the lining of the spinal cord and brain (bacterial meningitis).

Hemorrhage: excessive bleeding due to illness or injury.

Hemorrhoids: enlarged (varicose) veins, also known as piles, found in the anal area. They cause pain, itching, and bleeding, especially when the affected person also has constipation.

Hepatitis: inflammation of the liver caused by viruses and other organisms, drugs, alcohol, poisons, or other agents. The two major types of viral hepatitis are hepatitis A, which is spread by ingestion of contaminated substances, and hepatitis B, which is transmitted by contact with contaminated blood or blood products or via sexual transmission.

Hepatitis A virus: see: Hepatitis.

Hepatitis associated antigen: see Australian antigen.

Hepatitis B antigen: a substance in blood that indicates the presence of hepatitis B infection.

Hepatitis B core antigen: a substance found in the infected liver cells of patients who have hepatitis B.

Hepatitis B core antibody: a substance found in the blood of a person in the early stage of active hepatitis B infection.

Hepatitis B immunoglobulin: a substance containing antibodies to hepatitis B. If given to persons who have been exposed to this disease, they may avoid contracting the infection.

Hepatitis B virus: the virus that causes hepatitis B infection.

Hernia: protrusion of an organ through the tissues that contain it.

Herpes genitalis (type 2): a viral infection caused by type 2 of the herpes simplex virus, which is usually transmitted via sexual contact; causes genital lesions that may be painful, pustular, and may cause fever and swelling of the surrounding lymph glands in the groin.

Herpes simplex (type 1): a viral infection caused by the herpes simplex virus. It produces fluid-filled blisters on the skin and lips, which may itch or burn.

Herpes zoster: a painful herpesvirus infection running along certain nerve pathways; also known as shingles.

Heterophil antibody test: a test using sheep red blood cells to diagnose infectious mononucleosis.
Normal values: in serum, a titer of less than 1.56.

Hexosaminidase A and B: enzymes; a test is done on venous blood in adults, umbilical cord blood in newborns, or amniotic fluid in the fetus, to determine the level of the enzyme. A deficiency may indicate the presence of Tay-Sachs disease or Sandhoff disease. (See Tay-Sachs disease and Sandhoff disease.)
Normal values: 5.0-12.9 U/L (hexosaminidase A constitutes half to three-quarters of the total amount of this enzyme).

Hiatal hernia: a type of hernia in which the stomach protrudes through a weakened portion of the diaphragm; may cause ulcer-like symptoms.

High density lipoprotein cholesterol: a blood fat fraction that helps remove fatty deposits from tissues and blood vessels.
Normal values: more than 30-70 mg/dL.

High voltage electrophoresis: a laboratory method for studying types and quantities of certain biological substances such as blood.

Hinton test: a blood test for syphilis.
Normal value: in serum, negative.

His bundle: a group of heart muscle fibers that transmit electrical impulses from the upper chambers (atria) to the lower chambers (ventricles) to produce contraction of the ventricles.

Histamine test meal: a procedure done to determine the presence or absence of acid in the stomach. The stomach is emptied of all contents by tubal aspiration, histamine is given to stimulate gastric secretions, and gastric fluid samples are collected at 10- or 15-minute intervals for 1/2 to 1 hour.
Normal values:
mean, 11.8 mEq/hr;
high-normal limit, 18.7 mEq/hr.

Histoplasma agglutinins: agglutinins associated with fungal lung infection.
Normal values: in serum, a titer of less than 1 : 8.

Histoplasmin skin test: a test done to determine past infection with *Histoplasma capsulatum*, a fungus spread by the feces of infected birds, bats, or fowl. The chemical histoplasmin produced by the fungus is injected under the skin. Past or active infection produces a raised area on the skin within 24 to 48 hours.

Histoplasmosis: an infection caused by the organism *Histoplasma capsulatum*, which may produce respiratory disease or generalized (systemic) infection.

HIV antibody: a substance produced by the body's immune system to fight off infection by the AIDS virus. HIV antibodies found in a person's blood prove that he or she is infected with the AIDS virus.

HIV antibody test: a test for AIDS virus (HIV) antibodies. (See Enzyme-linked immunosorbent assay [ELISA].)

HIV disease: AIDS.

HIV negative: refers to a negative test result for the HIV (AIDS) virus or HIV antibodies, indicating the person does not have HIV infection.

HIV positive: refers to a positive test result for the HIV (AIDS) virus or HIV antibodies, indicating the person has HIV infection.

HIV wasting syndrome: a condition in which an HIV-infected person loses a substantial amount of weight due to lack of appetite, general debility, and diarrhea.

Hodgkin's disease: a cancerous disease of the lymph glands, spleen, liver, bone marrow, and certain other tissues. Fever, sweating, weakness, weight loss, and anemia are among the principal symptoms.

Homogentisic acid: an acid present in urine in alkaptonuria, a rare metabolic disease.
Normal value: in urine, negative.

Homovanillic acid: a product of normal metabolism; elevated urine levels may indicate various tumors of the adrenal gland.
Normal values: in urine after 24-hr collection, less than 15 mg.

Hookworm disease: intestinal infestation by parasitic worms that fasten themselves to the lining of the intestines and suck the victim's blood, sometimes causing anemia. The disease is prevalent in Asia, Africa, Central and South America, and in poor rural areas of the southern United States. Poor hygiene contributes to the problem.

Hormone: a chemical, produced by certain cells or organs of the body, that specifically regulates various physical processes.

Host: an animal or plant that supports a parasite.

Human chorionic gonadotropin (HCG): a hormone produced by cells of placental origin. High levels usually indicate pregnancy; very high levels may indicate multiple pregnancy or, in a nonpregnant woman, point to a gynecologic problem.
Normal values: less than 3 mU/mL.

Human chorionic somatropin: see Human placental lactogen (hPL).

Human growth hormone (hGH): a hormone secreted by the pituitary gland. Blood levels provide a measure of pituitary function.
Normal values: in serum, less than 10 ng/mL.

Human immunodeficiency virus (HIV): the virus responsible for causing acquired immunodeficiency syndrome (AIDS); formerly called human T-lymphotropic virus (HTLV III).

Human leukocyte antigen typing: a tissue typing process used to ascertain compatibility of tissues or fluids between one person and another prior to performing a tissue or organ transplant. The process is also used to determine paternity.

Human papillomavirus: the virus that causes genital warts. See: Genital warts.

Human placental lactogen (hPL) (human chorionic somatropin): a hormone of placental origin. Abnormal levels may indicate a possible multiple pregnancy, fetal distress, or a disease condition.
Normal values:
 in pregnant women,
  at 5-27 weeks, less than 4.6 µg/mL
  at 28-31 weeks, 2.4-6.1 µg/mL
  at 32-35 weeks, 3.7-7.7 µg/mL
  at 36 weeks to delivery, 5-8.6 µg/mL
 *pregnant women who have diabetes mellitus may have higher levels at term
 in nonpregnant women, less than 0.5 µg/mL
 in men, less than 0.5 µg/mL

Human T-lymphotropic retrovirus: AIDS virus.

Hyaline membrane disease: a disease seen mainly in premature infants, who may lack a substance, called surfactant, that stabilizes the air sacs in the lung. Without surfactant, the air sacs collapse, causing respiratory distress; also called infant respiratory distress syndrome.

Hydrocortisone: see Cortisol.

Hydrogen breath test: a diagnostic procedure done to determine lactose (milk sugar) intolerance by analyzing the amount of hydrogen present in exhaled breath. Excess hydrogen indicates lactose deficiency.

11-Hydroxyandrosterone: a sex hormone secreted by the testes and adrenal glands.
   Normal values:
      in urine after 24-hr collection,
         in men, 0.1-0.8 mg
         in women, 0.0-0.5 mg

α-Hydroxybutyric dehydrogenase: an enzyme in blood that may be elevated after tissue damage, such as occurs in heart attack.
   Normal values: in serum, 0-180 mU/mL (30°C), can vary with test method.

17-Hydroxycorticosteroids: a group of hormones, including cortisol and others, secreted by the cortex (outer layer) of the adrenal glands; urine levels are measured as a test of adrenal function and to diagnose hypo- or hyperadrenalism.
   Normal values:
      in urine,
         in men, 3-9 mg/24 hr
         in women, 2-8 mg/24 hr
         lower in children.
      After injection of 25 USP units ACTH, level is 2 to 4 times higher.

11-Hydroxyetiocholanolone: a sex hormone secreted by the testes and adrenal glands.
Normal values: in urine after 24-hr collection,
in men, 0.2-0.6 mg
in women, 0.1-1.1 mg

5-Hydroxyindoleacetic acid: an end product of serotonin metabolism. Serotonin normally constricts blood vessels and transmits nerve impulses, but also produces flushing, rapid heart beat, asthma, diarrhea, and other symptoms when present in abnormally high levels, as in certain tumors. It is elevated in the urine of patients with carcinoid syndrome, a condition produced by a type of tumor found in the appendix or other parts of the lower intestinal tract, and sometimes in the lungs.
Normal values:
as serotonin in whole blood, 0.05-0.20 µg/ml;
in urine after 24-hr collection, less than 9 mg.

Hydroxyproline: an amino acid; elevated levels are found in the urine in bone disease and certain inherited conditions such as Marfan's syndrome.
Normal values: in urine after 24-hr collection, 10-75 mg.

5-Hydroxytryptamine (serotonin): a substance in blood and tissues that constricts blood vessels and transmits nerve impulses; it is elevated in the urine in carcinoid syndrome, a condition produced by a type of tumor found in the appendix or lower intestinal tract, and sometimes in the lungs.
Normal values: in urine, 0.05-0.20 µg/ml.

Hyperbaric oxygen: greater than atmospheric concentration of oxygen, administered in a pressurized chamber to help heal skin grafts, and treat soft tissue infections, burns, and other conditions.

Hypercholesterolemia: excess cholesterol in the blood and tissue cells.

Hyperglycemia: an elevated blood sugar level, usually due to diabetes mellitus.

Hyperimmune: being unusually rich in antibodies; having greater than usual degree of immunity.

Hyperparathyroidism: excessive secretion of hormone by the parathyroid glands, resulting in loss of calcium from the bones, increased calcium levels in blood, formation of kidney stones, and various other complications.

Hypersensitivity (allergy): excessive sensitivity of tissues to substances or other stimuli inside or outside the body.

Hypertension: high blood pressure. Contributing factors include tension or excitement, obesity, smoking, heredity, kidney disease, and cardiovascular disease. High blood pressure usually develops in middle age, but may occur in younger people, especially those who are obese and do not exercise.

Hypertensive, arteriosclerotic: refers to a person who has high blood pressure and hardening of the arteries.

Hyperthermia: greatly increased body temperature, resulting from illness, an impaired body heat-regulating mechanism, certain medications, and other causes.

Hyperthyroidism: enlargement of and excess secretion of hormones by the thyroid gland. Elevated thyroid hormone levels in the blood cause an increase in the metabolic rate, nervousness, weight loss, increased heart rate, goiter, and other complications.

Hypertonic saline test: a test performed to find out whether excessive thirst is caused by the condition known as diabetes insipidus or by psychologic factors; also known as Carter-Robbins test and Hickey-Hare test.

Normal values: in urine, flow decreases considerably and urine osmolality increases immediately following intravenous infusion of saline solution or within 30 min after infusion has been stopped.

Hypertonic solution: a solution that has a higher osmotic pressure than a standard (reference) solution.

Hyperventilation: rapid, deep breathing, caused by excitement, anxiety, or other factors, that lowers the carbon dioxide content of the blood. Symptoms include dizziness, confusion, faintness, and muscle cramps.

Hypoglycemia: abnormally low blood sugar levels, which may be caused by excessive insulin secretion or intake, fasting, certain drugs or foods, or disease.

Hypoparathyroidism: a condition caused by damage to or removal of one or more of the parathyroid glands, which results in decreased secretion of parathyroid hormone. Consequences include lowered blood calcium levels and neuromuscular excitability that appears as tetany (muscle spasms and cramps).

Hypotension: low blood pressure.

Hypothermia: abnormally low body temperature caused by illness or exposure to cold, or induced, as for heart or brain surgery or to treat a high fever.

Hypothyroidism: reduced secretion of hormones by the thyroid gland caused by removal of the thyroid, iodine or other drug therapy, disease, or endocrine deficiency. It may occur in infants as a congenital syndrome called cretinism.

Hypotonic solution: one that has a lower osmotic pressure than a standard (reference) solution.

Hysterogram: an X-ray of the uterus after injection of contrast medium into the uterine cavity.

Hysterosalpingography: an X-ray of the uterus and fallopian tubes after injection of contrast medium.

Hysteroscopy: a procedure that allows direct visual examination of the uterus with a tubular instrument (endoscope) for diagnostic or treatment purposes.

I

Idiopathic thrombocytopenic purpura: a blood disease of unknown cause. Symptoms include skin hemorrhage, i.e., inadequate clotting of blood following small cuts, surgery, or other injury due to insufficient platelets in the blood.

Image intensifier: electronic equipment used in Xray studies that allows fluoroscopy to be performed with a lower dose of radiation, yet produces a brighter, more detailed image than is possible with a conventional fluoroscopy screen. The image intensifier also allows the use of closed-circuit television to film the process being studied.

Immune: protected against a given infection or disease process.

Immune bodies: antibodies that fight infection or agents foreign to the body.

Immune globulin: a blood protein fraction that contains antibodies.

Immune serum: serum that has immune properties (contains antibodies).

Immunity: resistance to disease or infection.

Immunity, acquired: immunity achieved sometime after birth.

Immunity, active: long-term ability of the cells to protect the body against a new infection, as a result of vaccination that stimulates development of specific antibodies.

Immunity, passive: temporary immunity conferred by injection or ingestion of prepared material containing antibodies against a specific disease or infection.

Immunodeficiency diseases: diseases caused by a deficiency in the body's protective immune system against foreign organisms. As a result, the body becomes susceptible to infection and other illnesses such as cancer.

Immunodiffusion: a laboratory technique used to detect the type and quantity of a substance, such as an abnormal immunoglobulin, for which an antibody is available.

Immunoelectrodiffusion: a laboratory technique similar to immunodiffusion, but speeded up by applying an electric current during the process.

Immunofluorescence: a laboratory procedure using fluorescein-labeled antibodies that aid in detecting antigens and the diagnosis of infectious diseases.

Immunofluorescent antibody: an antibody-tagging technique that uses a fluorescent stain (fluorescein) to detect infectious diseases and other illnesses.

Immunoglobulins (Ig) A, D, E, G, and M: a family of blood protein fractions, each with one or more specific functions. IgA is protective against vital and bacterial infections, and may cause transfusion reactions. The functions of IgD are not yet understood, although IgD can be isolated. IgE has a prominent role in allergic reactions, such as asthma or skin rash. IgG and IgM fight infection.
  Normal values:
    in serum:
      IgA, 60-330 mg/dL
      IgD, 0.5-3.0 mg/dL
      IgE, less than 500 ng/ML
      IgG, 550-1900 mg/dL
      IgM, 45-145 mg/dL

Immunohematology: the study of antigen-antibody reactions and their effects on blood.

Immunology: the science of immunity.

Immunosuppression: reduced ability of the body's immune system to function adequately in warding off illness.

Impedance plethysmography: occlusive impedance phlebography. A test done with special equipment that uses external electrodes and an inflatable pressure cuff (wrapped around the thigh) to detect blood clots or a risk for developing blood clots in each leg. The test can also assess the possibility of such clots in the lungs. The graphs obtained from the blood volume-measuring machine (plethysmograph) are then interpreted to obtain the results of the test. A slow rise or drop may indicate a blocked vein.
  Normal values: a noticeable rise on cuff inflation; a quick drop on cuff deflation

Impetigo: a skin infection, primarily affecting the face and extremities, that occurs most frequently in babies and small children. It's usually caused by Staphylococcus or Streptococcus bacteria. Red skin areas change to blisters that open and become covered with yellow crusts.

Impotence, organic: inability to have a penile erection due to a physical cause such as a circulatory disturbance.

Impotence, psychogenic: inability to have a penile erection caused by one or more underlying psychologic problems.

In vitro: refers to a laboratory test or other procedure conducted in a test tube or other laboratory dish.

In vitro fertilization: an artificial insemination technique in which an egg (ovum) is removed from a woman, and placed in a laboratory dish with sperm from the husband or a sperm donor. The fertilized egg is then implanted in the woman's uterus to start a pregnancy.

In vivo: refers to a laboratory test or other procedure conducted on a human or animal body.

Incision and drainage: a treatment method in which an abscess or other infected area is opened to allow release of pus and other abnormal materials and fluids.

Inclusion bodies: variously shaped bodies (particles) that occur in cells occupied by viruses.

Incompatibility: a state in which two substances cannot be mixed without one of them being changed or destroyed.

Increased intracranial pressure: a dangerous condition that may occur with certain diseases such as a tumor of the brain, or after a head injury. Pressure inside the brain increases as it expands due to tissue growth or blood or fluid build-up. The brain becomes compressed inside the skull, and measures to relieve the pressure must be taken promptly to avoid life-threatening brain damage.

Incubation period: the time between exposure to infection and the first symptoms of illness.

Incubator: a cabinet heated to a temperature that is kept constant to allow cultures of bacteria to grow; or a temperature-regulated apparatus for housing premature babies.

Indican: a substance excreted in urine. Elevated levels may indicate that the patient is on a high-protein diet or suffering from gastrointestinal disease.
Normal values: in urine after 24-hr collection, 10-20 mg

Indirect antiglobulin test: see: Indirect Coomb's test.

Indirect Coomb's test: a blood test done to cross-match blood and detect the cause of a transfusion reaction, and for various other purposes.

Infant respiratory distress syndrome: (transient tachypnea of the newborn) inability of the newborn infant's lungs to adequately handle normal respiratory functions, usually due to the immaturity of the lungs; seen especially in premature infants. Sometimes called neonatal wet lung syndrome. Symptoms include heavy breathing and inadequate oxygen intake caused by a delay in the reabsorption of lung fluid during fetal life.

Infection: a disease that results from invasion of the body by disease-causing microorganisms that multiply and produce injurious effects.

Infectious: pertaining to an infection that can be transmitted.

Infectious hepatitis: inflammation of the liver caused by an infectious organism such as a virus.

Infectious mononucleosis: a usually mild viral disease common among young people. Symptoms include fever, sore throat, swollen lymph glands, headache, and fatigue. More severe cases may affect the spleen and liver.

Infiltrate: a foreign substance introduced in tissue.

Inflammation: tissue reaction to an injury or irritant; symptoms include redness, heat, and pain.

Inflatable penile prosthesis: a surgically implanted device in the penis of men who suffer from impotence, which enables them to have sexual intercourse.

Influenza: a viral infection of the respiratory tract with symptoms that include fever, headache, sore throat, chills, cough, fatigue, and lack of appetite. Influenza is generally mild, but may affect the elderly or chronically ill more severely. The disease may occasionally become very virulent and spread as an epidemic across a large geographic area, country, or continent.

Inoculation: the introduction of infectious material or microbes into the body, usually to stimulate the development of immunity.

Insomnia: difficulty or inability to sleep at night.

Inspection, palpation, percussion, auscultation: processes used by health professionals during a physical examination. Inspection: Looking over a person's body for signs of disease or abnormality. Palpation: Feeling a person's chest, back or other body part. Percussion: Tapping certain body areas. Auscultation: Listening for heart sounds with a stethoscope.

Insulin: a protein hormone secreted by the pancreas that regulates carbohydrate metabolism.
> *Normal values:*
> in serum after a 12-hr fast, 5-30 μU/mL;
> in serum after glucose is administered, insulin rises to above 200 μU/mL within 4 hr. (This test cannot be done on a patient receiving insulin injections for treatment of diabetes.)

Insulin-dependent diabetes mellitus: see Diabetes mellitus.

Insulin shock: a condition usually seen in insulin-dependent diabetic patients who have taken too much insulin or have not eaten enough food to balance the amount of insulin injected. It also may occur in diabetic patients who are not well stabilized or in those who are ill or injured. Blood sugar drops to a very low level, resulting in such symptoms as tremors, a cold sweat, dizziness, and weakness. Coma may follow unless orange juice, sugar, candy, or specific medical management is provided to neutralize the excess insulin.

Insulin tolerance test: a test done on blood to determine certain hormonal functions, such as growth hormone secretory capacity and pituitary or adrenocortical insufficiency.

Normal values: blood glucose returns to 50% of normal fasting levels within 10-30 min after a calculated dose of crystalline zinc insulin is injected, and to normal levels within 90-120 min after the injection.

Intake and output: a measurement of fluids taken in versus fluids put out via urine, drainage of body fluid, or vomiting. Done to assess whether intake and output are balanced.

Intercurrent infection: an infection that develops in a person who already has another disease or infection.

Interferon: a protein released by cells invaded by viruses to inhibit viral multiplication.

Intermittent positive pressure breathing: a process wherein a ventilation machine uses alternately positive and negative pressure to aid a person with respiratory problems.

International unit (International system of units, SI): a system that standardizes measures of weight and volume in countries throughout the world.

Intestinal obstruction: a condition in which normal passage of intestinal contents is blocked by a tumor, by twisting or shifting of the intestines, or by a hernia or post-surgical adhesions. Symptoms include intense pain, constipation, vomiting, weakness, a gurgling noise in the bowels, and sometimes shock.

Intra-arterial digital subtraction angiography: a technique used to diagnose blood vessel abnormalities such as obstruction, closure, and others. The technique involves injection of contrast material into an artery, then using a computer and video terminal to produce an image of the area being examined.

Intracranial pressure: the pressure on the brain inside the skull.

Intraocular lens: an artificial lens for the eye, implanted in the eye's capsule after surgical extraction of the cloudy lens (cataract).

Intraocular pressure: pressure inside the eyeball.

Intrauterine device: a device inserted in the uterus for contraceptive purposes.

Intravascular coagulation test: a test done to detect internal coagulation of blood, a phenomenon that occurs in a number of blood coagulation disorders.
Normal values: in whole blood, no coagulation found.

Intravascular contrast echocardiography: injection of contrast material into the cardiovascular circulation to determine, with ultrasound, the direction and speed of blood flow in these areas.

Intravenous glucose tolerance test: a blood test done on diabetics, or to diagnose diabetes. The test involves an intravenous injection of glucose in the fasting state, then measuring the blood sugar level at specific intervals over a period of several hours.

Intravenous pyelogram: a radiographic record of the kidneys and urinary tract after intravenous injection of contrast medium to aid in visualization.

Intrinsic factor: see Unsaturated vitamin B_{12} binding capacity.

Inulin: a vegetable starch used in tests done to determine the adequacy of kidney function.

Inulin clearance: the rate at which the kidneys excrete inulin; tested to evaluate kidney function and diagnose muscle or liver diseases.
Normal values: in urine, 100-150 mL/min.

Iodine, butanol-extractable: iodine that can be separated from the plasma proteins by solvents such as butanol; it can be used as a measure of thyroid hormone levels in the blood to assess thyroid function.
Normal values: in serum, 3.5-6.5 µg/dL (results inaccurate if other forms of iodine given previously).

Iodine ring test: a test done on urine to detect the presence of bile.
Normal value: no change in the urine specimen's appearance.

Iron-binding capacity: a measure of the iron uptake and return in blood, in relation to the synthesis and breakdown of hemoglobin.
Normal values: in serum, 250-410 µg/dL.

Iron saturation, percent: the capacity of iron to saturate transferrin (an iron-binding substance); a measure of iron excess or deficiency. *Normal values:* in serum, 20-55%

Iron, total: a measure of the total blood level of iron.
Normal values: in serum, 75-175 µg/dL.

Irrigation and aspiration: cleaning and suctioning a wound or body cavity, to relieve accumulation of pus or other material, or to send a sample to the laboratory for examination.

Ischemia: a lack of blood in a given body area or organ; commonly caused by obstruction (narrowing or blockage of blood vessels) in that area due to abnormality or disease of the blood vessels.

Ischemic heart disease: illness that results from poor nourishment via the blood stream; develops as a result of narrowed or obstructed blood vessels that prevent adequate blood flow to the heart's tissues.

Isoantigen: an antigen that incites antibody production in members of the same species.

Isocitric dehydrogenase: an enzyme elevated in liver disease or placental problems of pregnancy.
Normal values: in serum, 50-300 U/mL.

Isoenzymes: enzymes that have slightly different chemical structures, but produce the same result, as the enzymes they resemble.

Isotonic solution: one that has the same osmotic pressure as a standard (reference) solution.

Isotope: one of a variety of forms in which a chemical element can appear. Isotopes of an element are identical in number of protons and electrons in each atom, but differ in mass number (total number of protons and neutrons in each atom's nucleus), and therefore have different properties.

J

Jaundice: a state in which the skin and other body parts turn yellowish due to elevated blood levels of bilirubin.

Joint range of motion: the measurement of a joint's ability to move through its arc, to assess and preserve the joint's capacity following injury or illness, and during the aging process.

Juvenile rheumatoid arthritis: an inflammatory disease of children that affects the joints of the fingers, wrists, feet, and sometimes other areas; also known as Still's disease. The joints become swollen, painful, and difficult to move. While rheumatoid arthritis is usually a long-term condition in adults, many children outgrow it.

K

Kaposi's sarcoma: a type of cancer in earlier times seen primarily in older men. Today it most often develops in a somewhat different form in male AIDS patients, with lesions on the skin or in various internal organs such as the gastrointestinal tract or the lungs.

Karyotyping: analysis of chromosomes; performed on fetal cells obtained by amniocentesis to detect the sex and various genetic factors or diseases of the unborn child. Karyotyping is also performed on children and young adults to detect genetic abnormalities and diseases.

Keep vein open: a term used in a hospital that indicates the need for a continuous intravenous infusion (usually using normal saline solution). Purpose: To allow immediate access if intravenous medication is required for emergency or other treatment purposes.

Kelling's test: a test done to detect the presence of lactic acid in the stomach. Lactic acid is normally seen in the stomach only in abnormal conditions.
  Normal value: no change, or very slight change in color of gastric fluid to which ferric chloride and water have been added. (Lactic acid produces a greenish-yellow color.)

Ketoacidosis: a serious condition found mainly in persons who have poorly controlled diabetes mellitus. Ketoacidosis occurs when there is a build-up of fatty acids (ketone bodies) in blood that are not properly metabolized due to an excess of blood sugar. Symptoms include lack of appetite, nausea, vomiting, and if allowed to continue untreated, coma and death.

11-Ketoandrosterone: a sex hormone secreted by the testes and adrenal glands.

Normal values:
>   in urine,
>> in men, 0.2-1.0 mg/24 hr;
>> in women, 0.2-0.8 mg/24 hr.

11-Ketoetiocholanolone: a sex hormone secreted by the testes and adrenal glands.

Normal values:
>   in urine after 24-hr collection,
>> in men, 0.2-1.0 mg;
>> in women, 0.2-0.8 mg.

Ketone bodies: a group of compounds produced by fatty acid metabolism, found in blood and urine only when a metabolic disturbance is present.

Normal values:
>   in serum, negative
>   in urine, negative

17-Ketosteroids: a group of adrenal cortical hormones with altered blood and urine levels in Addison's disease, Cushing's syndrome, stress, and endocrine disorders associated with precocious puberty, feminization in men, and excessive hair growth.

Normal values:
>   in plasma,
>> less than 30 µg/dL in the morning;
>> less than 10 µg/dL in the evening.
>   in urine after 24-hr collection,
>> in men, 6-18 mg;
>> in women, 4-13 mg (decreases with age);
>> in children, 12-15 yr, 5-12 mg;
>> in children under 12 yr, less than 5 mg.
>   levels increase 50-100% after injection of ACTH.

Kidney stone: a condition in which some solid matter separates from the urine flowing through the kidney and forms a stone inside the kidney or elsewhere in the urinary tract. Stones vary greatly in size and may be excruciatingly painful. Small stones may pass out of the urinary tract along with urine. Larger ones may obstruct the urinary tract or cause damage during passage.

Killed virus: used to prepare certain vaccines.

Knee endoscopy: the use of an endoscope to inspect the interior of the knee joint, to diagnose a torn cartilage or other abnormality. See also Arthroscopy.

Knee jerk: a normal response of the knee muscles that occurs when the physician uses an instrument to strike the leg below the knee joint. This is done as part of a neurological examination to test reflexes.

Kolmer's test: a blood test for syphilis.

Kwashiorkor: a syndrome caused by severe protein deficiency, found primarily in infants and children in underdeveloped countries. Symptoms include weakness, edema, enteritis, distended abdomen, liver changes, impaired growth and development, and pigmentation changes of the skin and hair.

Kymography: a technique used to record graphically the motions of body organs, such as the heart and the great blood vessels.

L

Lactic acid: a monobasic acid, the end product of the metabolism of sugar. Blood levels of lactic acid are elevated in patients with lactic acidosis, diabetes, anemia, and leukemia; following excessive exercise; and in other abnormal conditions.

Normal values:
> in whole blood,
>> venous, 5-20 mg/dL;
>> arterial, 3-7 mg/dL.

Lactic dehydrogenase: an enzyme; elevated in blood and tissues in various diseases including myocardial infarction, cancer, and anemia; elevated in CSF in various conditions, including stroke and meningitis.

Normal values:
> in serum, 200-600 U/mL, or up to 250 IU/mL;
> in CSF, approximately 1/10 of serum level.

Lactic dehydrogenase isoenzymes: a variety of molecular forms of lactic dehydrogenase; the pattern of distribution of the various isoenzymes (separated by electrophoresis) can help diagnose heart and liver disease.

Normal values: in serum,
> anode,
>> LDH_1, 17-27%
>> LDH_2, 27-37%
>> LDH_3, 3-8%
>> LDH_4, 0-5%

Lactose: a sugar excreted in urine. Its levels are elevated in late pregnancy, during lactation, and in certain rare metabolic diseases.
Normal values: in urine after 24-hr collection, 12-40 mg.

Lactose tolerance: the capacity of the body to handle lactose/glucose metabolism.

Normal values: in serum following ingestion of lactose, serum glucose changes are measured, and are comparable to those seen in a glucose tolerance test.

Laparoscopy: a procedure that employs an instrument called a laparoscope to look inside the abdomen to detect a number of possible abnormal conditions of the pelvic organs and their cause(s) such as inflammation, cysts, ectopic pregnancy, an abscess, adhesions, or pelvic pain. The laparoscope is inserted via a small abdominal incision, after local or general anesthesia has been administered.

Laryngitis: inflammation of the voice box (larynx). May cause hoarseness, sore throat, cough, and difficulty swallowing.

Laryngoscopy: examination of the larynx and the upper portion of the trachea with a laryngoscope to diagnose a tumor or other abnormality or to remove a foreign body.

Laryngotracheobronchitis: inflammatory condition caused by irritation or infection that involves the voice box (larynx), windpipe (trachea), and the bronchi (air sacs between the trachea and the lungs that store air).

Laser: a high-intensity light source used to excise tissue, thereby avoiding more traumatic surgical procedures.

Last menstrual period: the date of the start of a pregnant woman's most recent menstrual period, used to calculate the expected date of delivery.

Latex fixation test: a blood test to detect various antibodies and factors indicative of such conditions as rheumatoid arthritis, lupus erythematosus, dermatomyositis, and chronic infections.

Lead: a metallic element and normal blood constituent that can be toxic if ingested. If blood or urine levels are elevated, lead poisoning is likely.

Normal values:

in whole blood, less than 25 µg/dL

(60 µg/dL or more is considered toxic)

in urine after 24-hr collection, less than 80 µg

Lead apron, lead shield: a protective apron or device made of lead, worn by X-ray technicians, radiologists, and patients as protection against radiation during X-ray procedures.

Lecithin : sphingomyelin ratio: the ratio of two components of amniotic fluid; found to be a predictor of fetal lung maturity.

Normal values: a titer of 2:1 or greater.

Legionnaire's disease: a severe form of pneumonia caused by the bacterium *Legionella pneumophila.*

Leprosy: see Hansen's disease.

Leptospira agglutinins: agglutinins found in blood of patient's with Weil's disease, an infectious type of jaundice caused by the *Leptospira* organism.

Leucine aminopeptidase test: a test performed on blood to detect whether a person has liver disease or a bone and joint disease.

Normal values:

in men, 80-200 Goldberg-Rutenberg units;

in women, 75-185 Goldberg-Rutenberg units.

Leukapheresis: a process in which blood is withdrawn from a vein, white blood cells are selectively removed in a cell-separating machine, and the remainder of the blood is reinfused in the donor. The white blood cells may be used for treatment, research, or other purposes.

Leukemia: a cancer that affects the blood-forming system, causing production of large numbers of abnormal white blood cells that invade organs such as the bone marrow, liver, and kidneys. The disease occurs in two forms: acute leukemia, which frequently attacks children, and chronic leukemia, a less severe form that more often affects elderly people.

Leukocyte alkaline phosphatase test: a blood test done to detect various diseases that stimulate the secretion of this enzyme, such as cirrhosis, polycythemia, and certain infections. It is also used to differentiate chronic myelogenous leukemia from leukemoid reactions. (Also known as the neutrophil alkaline phosphatase test.)
Normal values: in smear of fresh venous blood, 50-150 U.

Leukocytosis: an increase of white blood cells in the circulation.

Leukopenia: a decrease of white blood cells in the circulation.

Lipase: a pancreatic enzyme active in fat digestion; may be elevated in pancreatitis.
Normal values: in serum, 0-1.5 Cherry-Crandall units/mL.

Lipoproteins (lipid profile): fatty acid fractions found in blood; elevated in certain diseases such as atherosclerosis.
Normal values:
  in serum:
    total, 400-800 mg/dL;
      cholesterol, 150-200 mg/dL, less in young adults;
      triglycerides, 10-190 mg/dL;
      fatty acids, 9.0-15.0 mmol/L;
      phospholipids as phosphorus, 9-16 mg/dL;
      phospholipids, 150-380 mg/dL;
      neutral fat, 0-200 mg/dL;
      low-density lipoproteins (varies with age), less than 130 mg/dL;
      high-density lipoproteins, 35-80 mg/dL.

Lithium: a metallic element; lithium compounds are used to treat certain types of mental illness. Lithium serum levels must be carefully monitored during treatment to avoid toxicity.
Normal value: negative
Therapeutic levels: 0.5-1.5 mEq/L
Toxic levels: more than 2.0 mEq/L

Lithotripsy: a procedure performed to crush kidney or bladder stones in the urethra, bladder, or ureter by means of extracorporeal shock waves that pulverize the stones, often making surgery unnecessary.

Liver scan: a scan of the liver after intravenous injection of a radioactive substance, to detect tumor, abscess, or degeneration, shown by a lack of uptake of the radioactive substance.

Long-acting thyroid-stimulating hormone: an agent with a prolonged effect on the thyroid gland; found in the blood in various thyroid conditions.
Normal value: in serum, negative

Low blood pressure: blood pressure below average levels consistent with age.

Low-density lipoprotein: a fraction of blood fat that tends to promote lipid (fatty) deposits in tissues and blood vessels, which may lead to clogging of the vessels and cause cardiovascular disease.
Normal values: less than 130 mg/dL

Lumbar puncture: aspiration of fluid from the spinal canal through a needle, to diagnose stroke, infection, tumor, or other conditions, or to determine the extent of injury after head, neck, or back trauma.

Lung compliance test (static): a test that measures the elastic properties of the lungs. *Normal values:* 0.2 L/cm H_2O

Lung scan: (1) Perfusion scan: a scanning procedure involving intravenous injection of radioactive albumin and examination of lung structure and function, to diagnose pulmonary embolism. (2) Ventilation scan: a procedure in which the patient breathes in radioactive gas and the lungs are scanned for areas that don't receive air, or for other abnormalities.

Lupus erythematosus: an inflammatory disease that occurs in two forms. The discoid type usually produces butterfly-shaped, red skin lesions on the face. The more serious systemic type affects connective tissues and joints as well as the heart, lungs, and other organs.

Lupus erythematosus cell test: a test for a specific type of white blood cell, done in patients suspected of having lupus erythematosus. Such cells also occur in other diseases such as lupoid hepatitis and rheumatoid arthritis. *Normal values:* in venous blood, fewer than 2 LE cells/5-10 mL.

Luteinizing hormone: a hormone that originates in the anterior portion of the pituitary gland and controls various reproductive functions.
  Normal values: in serum,
    in men, less than 6-18 mU/mL;
    in Women,
      premenopausal, less than 25 mU/mL
      mid-cycle peak, more than 3x baseline value
      postmenopausal, more than 30 mU/mL.

Luteinizing hormone-releasing factor: a substance in blood that aids in the release of luteinizing hormone into the blood stream.

Lyme disease: a disease transmitted by ticks, that was originally identified in Lyme, Connecticut. Symptoms include reddish skin lesions and arthritis-like joint pains. In more severe cases, neurologic symptoms such as meningitis may complicate the illness. Occurs primarily in regions where deer, who carry the ticks, are abundant.

Lymph: fluid that collects in body tissues, then flows through lymph glands and lymphatic channels into the venous circulation.

Lymphadenopathy-associated virus: another name for the AIDS virus.

Lymphangiography: an X-ray study of lymph glands and lymphatic channels after injection of contrast medium.

Lymphocyte: a type of white blood cell, active in fighting off infections.

Lymphocyte transformation: a test done on blood to determine the presence of abnormalities of the immune system, exposure to agents that cause diseases such as malaria, or to assess compatibility factors between tissue transplant donors and recipients. Several different assays are used to determine the results of the test.
Normal values:
mitogen assay, stimulates index over 10;
antigen assay, stimulates index over 3;
mixed lymphocyte culture (MLC) assay, no response indicates D-locus antigen histocompatibility.

Lymphocytic leukemia: the abnormal increase of white blood cells consisting of lymphocytes.

Lymphogranuloma venereum: a sexually transmitted disease (infection) caused by *Chlamydia trachomatis*. Causes a variety of genital and other symptoms.

Lymphoid interstitial pneumonia: a type of pneumonia most often found in children under 13 years of age who have AIDS.

Lymphoma: a tumor consisting of lymph node tissue.

Lysozyme muramidase test: a test done on blood or urine to detect the presence of certain forms of leukemia and other disease conditions.

Normal values:
in blood, 2.8-8.0 μg/mL;
in urine, less than 2.0 μg/mL.

M

Macroglobulins, total: heavy serum globulins, elevated in diseases including cancer and infections.
Normal values: in serum, 70-430 mg/dL.

Macroscopic: visible to the naked cyc.

Magnesium: an essential body mineral, measured in blood and urine to indicate the adequacy of a variety of body functions, including those of muscles and nerves, and of body fluids. Deficiency may indicate malnutrition, glandular hyperactivity, or other abnormalities. Excess levels may indicate dehydration, or inadequate adrenal function.
Normal values:
in blood, 1.8-3.0 mg/dL;
in urine after 24-hr collection, 6.0-8.5 mEq.

Magnetic resonance angiography: a computerized imaging technique that enables the doctor to visualize and study the heart.

Magnetic resonance imaging: a procedure in which a scanning device uses a magnetic field together with radiofrequency energy that allows penetration of bone to visualize soft tissue to determine abnormal conditions of brain and spinal cord soft tissues. Such conditions as edema (swelling of tissues due to excessive fluid accumulation), tumors, and diseases such as multiple sclerosis may be diagnosed with this technique.

Malaria: a disease caused by *Plasmodium* protozoa, transmitted to humans by the bite of the Anopheles mosquito or blood from infected donors. Attacks may occur repeatedly, causing fever, chills, sweating, malaise, headache, and muscular pains. The disease is treated with drugs and prevented by elimination of mosquito breeding areas.

Malignant hyperthermia: an inherited condition whose symptoms are usually triggered by anesthesia. Symptoms include extremely high temperature and muscular rigidity.

Mammography: an X-ray technique used to examine breast tissue for tumors or other abnormalities, and to differentiate between benign and malignant growths.

Manometry: the measurement of pressures in various body parts.

Mantoux test: a skin test to detect the presence of, or exposure to, tuberculosis. *Normal value:* negative reaction if there is no disease or exposure.

Marasmus: debilitated condition caused by chronic malnutrition.

Marfan's syndrome: an inherited disorder that affects many body systems, such as the skeletal, respiratory, and cardiovascular; and the eyes.

Mass spectrometry: an ionizing technique that uses the mass of compounds to identify and quantitate them. Peptides, catecholamines, bile acids, and various drugs are analyzed by this method.

Maturity-onset diabetes of youth: a rare, relatively mild form of diabetes mellitus in children or young people.

Maximal acid output: see Gastric fluid.

Maximal breathing capacity: the amount of air a person can breathe per minute.

Maximal mid-expiratory flow: liters per second of air expelled from the lungs during forced exhalation; a test of air flow obstruction.

Maximal voluntary ventilation: see Maximal breathing capacity.

Mazzini's test: a blood test for syphilis. Normal value in serum: negative

Mean corpuscular hemoglobin (MCH): a measure of the average hemoglobin content per red blood cell.
Normal values: in whole blood, 27-31 pg/cell.

Mean corpuscular hemoglobin concentration (MCHC): a measure of hemoglobin concentration in the average red blood cell; expressed as a ratio of hemoglobin to volume of packed red cells.
Normal values: in whole blood, 32-36% of packed red blood cells.

Mean corpuscular volume (MCV): a measure of the average size of the red blood cells.
Normal values: in whole blood, 80-96 μ^3.

Measles (rubeola): an infectious vital disease that occurs mainly in children and young adults. Symptoms include fever, cold-like symptoms, headache, characteristic lesions in the mouth (Koplik spots), and a red rash on the body. Widespread vaccination of children has greatly reduced the incidence of this disease in the United States.

Mediastinoscopy: a test done to determine diseases and other abnormalities of the lungs. The test is performed under general anesthesia, with an instrument (endoscope) that permits visualization of the lungs and surrounding structures. Tissue specimens are obtained and examined after removal.

Melanin, qualitative: a urine test for melanin, a normal pigment found in urine in patients with malignant melanoma, a type of cancer.
Normal value: negative

Meniere's disease: a neurologic condition characterized primarily by dizziness, nausea, sometimes vomiting, and increasing deafness.

Meningitis: inflammation of the membranes (meninges) that surround the brain and spinal cord. May be caused by injury, irritation, infection, or other factors. Symptoms may include severe headache, fever, a stiff neck, and vomiting.

Meningococcal infection: one of the principal causes of meningitis. Meningococcus organisms (*Neisseria meningitidis*) may enter the bloodstream and cause meningococcemia, a generalized infection.

Menopause: the period during a woman's life when menstrual periods occur irregularly and finally cease. Also known as the climacteric, this condition generally starts between the ages of 45 and 50, and may last from several months to several years.

Metabolism: the physical and chemical changes in the body that are responsible for maintaining function and nutrition.

Metabolite: a product of metabolism.

Methemoglobin: a compound found in the blood following ingestion of nitrates, aspirin substitutes, and food preservatives.
Normal value: in whole blood, negative.

3-Methoxy-4-hydroxymandelic acid: an excretory product of the catecholamines (adrenaline and noradrenaline); tested in urine as an indirect measure of catecholamine levels. Elevated levels may raise the blood pressure, or indicate the presence of adrenal gland or nervous tissue tumors, and such conditions as muscular dystrophy and myasthenia gravis. Certain drugs, foods, stress, and exercise can also cause elevated levels of this substance.
Normal values:
> in urine after 24-hr collection,
>> in adults, 1.5-7.5 mg;
>> in infants, 83 μg/kg of body weight.

Microbe: a microscopic organism.

Microhemagglutination assay: a laboratory test done to diagnose syphilis.

Microscopic: invisible without the use of a microscope.

Microsomal antibody: see Thyroid antibodies.

Mid-stream catch urine specimen: a urine specimen collected during the middle of the urine flow, done after the urinary opening (meatus) has been carefully cleaned.

Migraine: intense headache, sometimes confined to one side of the head, often accompanied by nausea, vomiting, and visual symptoms. The cause is unknown, but may involve factors such as tension, changes in cerebral circulation, muscle spasm, or heredity.

Minimal inhibitory concentration (MIC), minimal bactericidal concentration (MBC): the lowest concentration in blood at which an antibiotic medication is effective against an infection. Venous blood, containing the infectious organism, is placed in a sterile tube and then inoculated into a liquid culture medium that contains several concentrations of antibiotic drug ranging from 100 μg/mL to as low as 0.195 μg/mL. The lowest concentration at which growth is arrested or the microorganism is killed is then reported, and this concentration is used to monitor the effects of further antibiotic treatment.

Minnesota Multiphasic Personality Inventory (MMPI): a test consisting of 550 statements to be interpreted by the subject; used in clinical psychology for overall personality evaluation and to determine the presence of various personality disorders, such as depression and schizophrenia.

Minute ventilation: the total amount of air exhaled from the lungs each minute (tidal volume multiplied by the respiratory rate per minute).

Mitral valve prolapse: incomplete closure of the leaflet (valve) that opens and shuts between the left upper chamber of the heart (atrium) and the lower chamber (ventricle) to allow blood to flow from the atrium to the ventricle. This flaw may result in some back-flow (regurgitation) of blood.

Mixed culture: a culture that contains two or more different strains of organisms.

***Molluscum contagiosum*:** a sexually transmitted disease caused by a DNA poxvirus. Causes a variety of genital and other symptoms.

Monoamine oxidase: an enzyme; it is inhibited by a group of drugs that are effective in the treatment of depression.

Monoamine oxidase inhibitor: drug used in treating depression.

Monoclonal antibody: antibodies that are made from a particular cell clone, all of which have similar molecules. They are used for various research and treatment purposes.

Monoclonal antibody test: a diagnostic procedure to detect the presence of certain tumors that secrete antigens picked up by monoclonal antibodies.

Mononucleosis: see Infectious mononucleosis.

Monospot test: see Heterophil antibody test.

Morbidity: the state of being ill.

Motility test: a test done to observe the motility of organisms in "hanging drop" suspensions or culture preparations.

Motor evoked potential: recording of the electrical properties of muscles such as in the arms or legs during their resting and active phases, to diagnose various muscle diseases.

Motor nerve conduction velocity: a measurement of the time taken by a nerve impulse to travel a specific length of the nerve path.

Motor neuron disease: progressive weakness and deterioration of muscle tissue, caused by degenerative nervous diseases such as amyotrophic lateral sclerosis.

Mucus: a translucent, gelatinous material; it is normally present in feces in small quantities, but when present in larger quantities indicates a bowel abnormality.
Normal values: in stool, negative or small amount.

Multi-drug-resistant tuberculosis: a type of tuberculosis that resists normally effective medications.

Multiple myeloma: a form of cancer in which the body develops plasma cell tumors that invade the bone marrow and weaken and destroy bony structures such as the ribs, spine, pelvis, and skull. Principal symptoms include pain and fracture of affected bones.

Multiple sclerosis (MS): a progressive disease in which hard, gray patches (scleroses) form on the nerve coverings in the brain and spinal cord, gradually disrupting transmission of nerve impulses. The disease progresses unevenly, and remissions, during which the patient appears to improve, are common. As the disease advances, activities such as walking become increasingly difficult.

Mumps: a contagious disease, usually contracted during childhood, caused by a virus transmitted in saliva. Symptoms include swelling of the parotid (saliva) glands behind each ear, headache, and fever. The testes, ovaries, or pancreas may also be affected.

Muscle biopsy: a diagnostic procedure in which small pieces of muscle are surgically removed and examined for the presence of disease.

Muscular dystrophy (MD): a hereditary disease that causes progressive weakness and wasting of muscle tissue.

Myasthenia gravis (MG): a neuromuscular disorder of unknown origin that weakens muscles by interfering with normal transmission of nerve impulses to muscle fibers. Certain drugs are helpful in counteracting muscular weakness and restoring function.

Mycobacterium avium-intracellulare: an organism generally seen when it causes opportunistic infection in an AIDS patient.

Mycobacterium tuberculosis: the organism that causes tuberculosis.

Mycophage: a fungal virus.

Mycosis: any disease caused by a fungus.

Mycosis fungoides: a fairly rare form of chronic lymphoma affecting the skin and internal organs.

Mycotoxin: a toxin produced by fungi.

Myelography: an X-ray study of the spinal cord after injection of contrast medium.

Myocardial infarction (MI): a heart attack; a potentially fatal condition in which a part of the heart muscle dies due to an interruption of its essential blood supply.

Myoglobin: a constituent of blood normally present in a tiny amount, elevations may indicate damage of the heart muscle after a heart attack (MI) or skeletal muscles following an injury.
Normal values:
> in urine after 24-hr collection,
>> qualitative, negative;
>> quantitative, less than 1.5 mg/L.

N

Nasogastric tube: a thin, flexible tube passed through the nose, esophagus, and into the stomach. The tube may be used to feed a person who cannot eat food by mouth; as part of postoperative management; to remove blood or other substances from the stomach; and to perform diagnostic procedures.

Necrosis: the death of cells or tissues caused by trauma, a burn, or disease.

Necrotizing fasciitis: a rare, severe infection caused by organisms including certain streptococcus organisms that attack and rapidly destroy skin and muscle tissue. Immediate antibiotic treatment is needed to control the infection and save the patient's life.

Necrotizing ulcerative gingivitis (Vincent's infection, trench mouth): an infection that causes ulcerous lesions of the gums with tissue destruction that may spread to other membranes in the mouth. May be caused by poor dental and mouth hygiene, stress, and other conditions such as nutritional deficiency, debilitating illness, and smoking.

Needle biopsy: a sample of body tissue or fluid obtained via aspiration with a syringe and needle.

Nephritis: inflammation of the kidneys from any of a variety of causes, most commonly streptococcal infections.

Nephrosis: malfunctioning of the kidneys that may occur in conjunction with nephritis or various other conditions. Swelling of tissues (edema) from fluid accumulation occurs because the kidneys are unable to regulate fluid balance in the body.

Nerve conduction studies: see Electromyogram.

Neuralgia: painful sensations along a nerve pathway.

Neurofibromatosis: a hereditary condition characterized by pigmented skin spots and tumors on the skin and nerves. As the tumors grow they may need to be removed surgically or treated with radiation.

Neuropathy: disease of nerve tissue; may occur as a result of other illness such as diabetes mellitus.

Neuroradiology: X-ray studies of the central nervous system, including the brain and spinal cord.

Neurosyphilis: syphilis that affects the brain or spinal cord; usually seen in the late stages of untreated syphilis.

Neutral fat: see under Fat, neutral.

Nitrogen, total: the nitrogen content of the feces; measured to detect such conditions as pancreatic insufficiency or impaired protein digestion.
   Normal values: in 24-hr specimen, 10% of intake or 1-2 g.

Nocturnal penile tumescence monitoring: a process used to determine, via one of several different methods, if a man is capable of having an erection.

Nocturnal polysomnography: a study of physiologic activities in sleep, done in a "sleep laboratory."

Nongonococcal urethritis: a sexually transmitted disease (infection) primarily caused by *Chlamydia trachomatis* and *Ureaplasma urealyticum*. May cause a variety of genital and other symptoms, or none.

Non-insulin-dependent diabetes mellitus (NIDDM) (type 2): see Diabetes mellitus.

Non-protein nitrogen: the nitrogen in the blood not appearing as protein; about half is normally present as urea. Blood levels can be measured to determine kidney function.
Normal values:
in serum or plasma, 20-35 mg/dL;
in whole blood, 25-50 mg/dL.

Non-rapid eye movement sleep: period of sleep during which no rapid eye movement occurs; about 75-80% of nighttime sleep.

Nonsteroidal anti-inflammatory drugs: medications containing no steroid ingredients that relieve and treat inflammatory conditions such as arthritis.

Norepinephrine: noradrenaline; a catecholamine hormone.
Normal values: in urine, less than 100 µg/24 hr.

Nosocomial infection: an infection acquired by a patient while in the hospital or other health-care facility.

Nuclear magnetic resonance: a new, noninvasive diagnostic method that uses magnetic forces to produce cross-sectional images of body structures; also called magnetic resonance imaging.

Nuclear medicine: a branch of medicine that uses radioisotopes in diagnostic and treatment procedures.

Nuclear scanning (radionuclide organ imaging): a diagnostic procedure in which a radioactive substance (radioisotope or radionuclide) is administered orally or by injection. A scanning device is then used to detect radioactivity in particular body areas. The size, shape, location, and function of body parts can then be recorded via a computer printout. The radioactive substance does not harm the patient.

Nucleic acids: chemical compounds, found in all living cells, that are responsible for the transmission of hereditary characteristics.

Nucleolus: a spherical body inside the cell's nucleus that participates in the multiplication and metabolism of the cell.

5-Nucleotidase: a nonlipid enzyme, elevated in some liver diseases, used to distinguish between certain liver and bone diseases.

Normal values: in serum, 3.5-12.7 mU/mL (37○C).

Nucleus: the central body of the cell that determines its functions.

O

Obstructive sleep apnea (Pickwickian syndrome): a respiratory problem that occurs during sleep, which involves intermittent sudden cessation of breathing. This may be caused by a variety of conditions such as an abnormality in the airway (nose, mouth, palate), obesity, and snoring.

Occult: hidden; obscure.

Occult blood: see Blood, occult.

Open reduction and internal fixation: an orthopedic surgical procedure done to set a broken bone; an incision is made at the site of the fractured bone, which is then immobilized and set in its normal position.

Operating room radiography: X-ray studies done in the operating room during a surgical procedure.

Ophthalmoscopy: a direct, visual examination of the interior structures of the eye with an ophthalmoscope, for diagnostic or other purposes.

Opportunistic infection: an infection acquired as a result of another condition that lowers the body's resistance to disease.

Opsonins: blood components that enable cells to fight off microorganisms that invade the body.

Oral contraceptive: a pill containing one or more female hormones, which prevents pregnancy when taken regularly and according to the physician's instructions.

Oral glucose tolerance test: see: Glucose tolerance test, oral.

Ornithine carbamoyl transferase: an enzyme found in the blood in increased levels in liver and certain other diseases.
Normal values: in serum, 8-20 mIU/mL.

Osmolality: the osmotic concentration of blood or urine; a measure of its physicochemical properties.
Normal values:
in serum, 280-295 mOsm/kg serum water;
in urine, 38-1400 mOsm/kg water.

Osmosis: the process by which fluid passes across a permeable membrane from a solution of lesser to a solution of greater concentration.

Osmotic fragility test: a blood test in which red blood cells are placed in a series of successively weaker salt solutions to detect the point at which hemolysis (breakdown of red blood cells) occurs from osmotic pressure difference. Abnormally fragile cells break down in stronger solutions.
Normal values: in 24 hrs at 37oC: hemolysis begins in 0.45-0.39% salt solution and is complete in 0.33-0.30% salt solution.

Osteoarthritis: degeneration of cartilage at the end portion of bones; also called degenerative joint disease. As bones rub against each other, pain, swelling, and stiffness result.

Osteomyelitis: an infection of bone and/or bone marrow.

Osteoporosis: a decrease in the amount of bone tissue, producing brittle, fragile bones that can result in fracture. Causes include inadequate nutrition, menopausal changes resulting in a lack of estrogen, certain illnesses, and lack of exercise.

Ova and parasites test: microscopic examination of feces for parasites such as worms or amoebae and their eggs (ova), to detect parasitic infection.

Oxalate: a test done on urine to detect a metabolic defect that may cause kidney stones and other kidney disorders.

Normal values: urine oxalate levels up to 40 mg/24 hr.

Oxygen: a gas forming about 21% of atmospheric air; essential to respiration.

Normal values:

in arterial whole blood, (see also Partial pressure of oxygen)

capacity, 16-24 vol%

content, 15-23 vol%

saturation, 94-100% of capacity

P

P wave: a section of an electrocardiogram tracing that indicates depolarization of the upper heart chambers (atria), which results in their contraction; used in diagnostic studies of the heart.

P24 antigen test (p24 antigen capture assay): a laboratory test that measures the protein p24, which is found in the core of the AIDS virus (HIV).

Pacemaker: an artificial device that provides electric stimulation to regulate the heartbeat; it can be either temporary or permanent. Current permanent pacemakers may last 8-10 years before requiring replacement.

Pacemaker installation fluoroscopy: fluoroscopic monitoring used to guide the insertion of a pacemaker.

Pancreas scan: a scan of the pancreas after intravenous injection of a radioactive substance, to diagnose a tumor, cyst, infection, or other abnormality.

Pandemic: an epidemic disease that affects a large area, possibly one or more entire continents.

Pap (Papanicolaou) smear: a microscopic examination of cells taken from different parts of the body, often the cervix and vagina, to detect abnormalities such as cancer, infection, and effects of irradiation, and to determine cellular hormonal activity.

Para-aminohippuric acid, sodium (clearance): the rate at which the kidneys remove this substance from the blood; measured to detect kidney damage or certain muscle diseases.
   Normal values: in serum, 600-700 mL/min; in 24-hr urine collection, 600-750 mL/min.

Paracentesis: the puncture and withdrawal of fluid from the abdominal cavity, usually to remove excessive fluid accumulated as a result of a disease process.

Parasite: an organism that survives by feeding on another.

Parathyroid hormone (parathormone) (PTH): a test done on blood to determine the level of this hormone. Abnormally high levels may increase the amount of calcium and decrease the phosphorus levels in the circulation.
> *Normal values:* (determined in conjunction with calcium levels),
>> Intact PTH, 210-310 pg/mL
>> N-terminal fraction, 230-630 pg/mL
>> C-terminal fraction, 410-1,760 pg/mL

Parkinson's disease: a chronic progressive illness that affects the brain, causing gradual loss of control over voluntary movements accompanied by tremor and muscle rigidity; also known as paralysis agitans and shaking palsy.

Paronychia: also known as a whitlow or felon, this condition involves inflammation of the tissues surrounding a fingernail or toenail, producing pain, swelling, and often pus.

Paroxysmal atrial tachycardia: a sudden increase in the heart rate to as much as 100-200 beats per minute. Symptoms include a fast, fluttering sensation in the chest, along with feelings of weakness, palpitations, low blood pressure, and shortness of breath.

Paroxysmal supraventricular tachycardia: see: Paroxysmal atrial tachycardia.

Paroxysmal tachycardia: an sudden increase in the heart rhythm that produces a very rapid heart rate.

Partial pressure of carbon dioxide (PCO_2): the portion of total gas pressure exerted by the carbon dioxide in blood; increased in certain respiratory conditions and in chest injuries, decreased in uncontrolled diabetes, liver or kidney disease, severe diarrhea, and during rapid breathing.

Normal values:
    in arterial blood, 35-45 mm Hg;
    in venous blood, 40-45 mm Hg.

Partial pressure of oxygen (PO_2): the portion of total gas pressure exerted by oxygen in its gas phase in equilibrium with blood; decreased in obstructive lung disease, asthma, heavy exercise, and certain blood diseases.

Normal values: in arterial blood, 75-100 mm Hg.

Partial thromboplastin time (PTT): a blood test to screen for coagulation (clotting) disorders such as hemophilia, or to monitor anticoagulant medication.

Normal values: in plasma, 60-85 sec (after addition of partial thromboplastin reagent and ionized calcium).

Passive immunity: temporary immunity conferred by injection or ingestion of prepared material containing antibodies against a specific disease.

Patch test: a skin test for sensitivity to a particular substance. A small amount of solution containing the substance in question is placed on the patient's arm and covered, and the skin is observed for a reaction a few days later.

Reaction evaluation: considered positive if the skin area becomes red, swollen, irritated, or develops blisters

Pathogen: any organisms, such as bacteria or viruses, that can cause disease.

Pathology: the science of disease.

Patient-controlled analgesia: pain relief controlled by the patient, usually provided following a surgical procedure. The process involves an intravenous infusion containing a predetermined amount of a pain drug, which the patient releases into his or her blood stream as needed.

Paul-Bunnell test: a blood test for heterophil antibodies, used to confirm the diagnosis of infectious mononucleosis. See also Heterophil antibody test.
Normal value: negative

Pediculosis pubis: a sexually transmitted disease (infection) caused by the crab louse. May cause various genital and other lesions.

Pelvic inflammatory disease (PID): infection of the structures of a woman's genital tract, primarily the fallopian tubes. PID generally occurs in sexually active younger women as a result of sexually transmitted diseases. It may sometimes occur after childbirth or abortion.

Pelvimetry: manual measurement or X-ray study of the pelvic bones to determine if the space is adequate for giving birth.

Penicillin hypersensitivity skin test: a test done to determine sensitivity (allergy) to penicillin. A highly dilute solution of penicillin is injected into the skin. If no allergic reaction occurs, it's safe to administer the drug.

Penicillinase-producing Neisseria gonorrhoeae: a gonorrheal infection caused by organisms containing a substance (penicillinase) that resists treatment with penicillin. A special type of penicillinase-resistant penicillin must be used to treat these cases.

Pentose: a type of sugar, elevated after ingestion of plums and cherries, and in certain rare diseases.
Normal values: in urine after 24-hr collection, 2-5 mg/kg.

Peptic ulcer: an open, inflamed sore that occurs in the stomach or duodenum, often in people who suffer from frequent stress. Pain is usually worse when stomach is empty; may feel better by eating or drinking.

Percussion and auscultation: tapping various body areas such as the front and back of the chest, and listening to organs such as the heart or lungs with a stethoscope, usually during a physical examination.

Percutaneous transhepatic cholangiography: an X-ray technique in which dye is injected through the liver into the bile duct to detect obstruction.

Percutaneous transluminal coronary angioplasty: a procedure done to dilate narrowed areas in the heart's major blood vessels. A small, balloon-tipped catheter is passed into the obstructed vessel, and the balloon is inflated to widen the vessel's diameter.

Perfusion scan: see Lung scan.

Perfusion test, acid (Bernstein test): a test performed on a patient's esophagus (gullet) to determine whether a complaint of chest pain is due to a possible heart problem or inflammation of the esophagus. The test is done by passing a thin tube (catheter) through the patient's nose, behind the mouth, and into the esophagus. Saline and acid solutions then drip into the esophagus, and the patient is asked to report any painful or burning sensation, as well as the location.
Normal value: no pain or burning sensation felt during the test

Pericardial fluid: the fluid contained in the membranous sac surrounding the heart. In certain diseases, the amount of fluid may increase and press on the heart.

Pericardiocentesis: a test performed on fluid removed from the sac that surrounds the heart. Under local anesthesia, the fluid is withdrawn from the pericardial space (the area surrounding the heart) with a sterile needle, to determine causes of excessive build-up in the sac.

Perinatal transmission: transmission of an infection by a pregnant woman to her fetus before birth, while giving birth, or within a short time after birth.

Peripheral arteriovenography: an X-ray of the arteries and veins in the peripheral parts of the body, such as the arms and legs, following injection of contrast medium into the vein.

Peripheral vascular disease: inadequate blood supply to the extremities caused by disorders of the arteries, veins, and lymphatic vessels that supply the arms and legs.

Peritonitis: inflammation of the membrane that lines the abdominal cavity and covers the abdominal organs; peritonitis may occur following infection or trauma or as a complication of diseases of the internal organs.

Pernicious anemia: a disease, often occurring in middle or old age, in which red blood cells fail to develop normally because of vitamin B_{12} deficiency. Symptoms include fatigue, pallor, weakness, loss of appetite, dizziness. Vitamin B_{12} injections control condition.

Persistent generalized lymphadenopathy: enlarged lymph nodes often seen in people with HIV (AIDS virus) infection.

Pertussis (whooping cough): a highly communicable disease characterized by severe cough paroxysms that end in a sound like a whoop.

Petri dish: a covered glass dish used in the laboratory to grow microorganisms.

pH: the hydrogen ion concentration (degree of acidity or alkalinity) of a substance. The neutral point is pH 7; values below 7 indicate acidity; values above 7 indicate alkalinity. Maximum acidity is pH 0; maximum alkalinity is pH 14.
Normal values:
in whole arterial blood, 7.35-7.45;
in urine, 4.6-8.0.

Phage typing: identification of bacteria by testing their susceptibility to bacterial viruses.

Phagocyte: a cell that consumes bacteria and other foreign matter.

Pharyngitis: inflammation of the pharynx, the upper portion of the throat.

Phenobarbital/phenytoin serum levels: the concentrations of these drugs in the serum; monitored to maintain blood levels adequate to control seizures but not high enough to cause toxic reactions.
Therapeutic values: 10-30 μg of each drug per mL of whole blood.

Phenol coefficient: a measure of disinfectant activity of a given chemical in relation to carbolic acid (phenol).

Phenolsulfonphthalein: a dye used in kidney function tests. Urine levels are measured at regular intervals after injection of 6 mg, to test the excretory capacity of the kidney tubules. Rate of excretion is decreased in kidney and some urinary tract diseases, increased in some liver diseases.
Normal values: after inj 1 mL PSP intravenously,
after 15 min, 25% or more of dye excreted;
after 30 min, 40% or more of dye excreted;
after 120 min, 50% or more of dye excreted.

Phenylalanine: an amino acid that accumulates in excessive amounts in phenylketonuria, an inherited enzyme deficiency disease that causes mental retardation if not diagnosed and treated soon after birth.
Normal values: in serum,
in adults, less than 3.0 mg/dL;
in term newborns, 1.2-3.5 mg/dL.

Phenylketonuria: see Guthrie bacterial inhibition assay.

Phenylpyruvic acid: an intermediate product of phenylalanine metabolism; present in the urine in certain metabolic diseases of the newborn. *Normal value:* in urine, qualitative, negative.

Phlebitis: inflammation of a vein.

Phonocardiography: a procedure in which a transducer is applied to the chest to identify abnormal heart sounds in such conditions as heart valve disease and heart enlargement; frequently done in combination with apexcardiography and electrocardiography.

Phosphatase, acid (total): an enzyme present in kidney, serum, semen, and the prostate gland. The enzyme level is increased in serum in trauma or cancer of the prostate, and various other conditions; also used to screen for the presence of semen in rape cases. *Normal values:* 0.1-1 Bodansky units/mL

Phosphatase, alkaline (total): an enzyme present especially in teeth, bone, plasma, kidney, and intestine. The serum level is increased in certain bone, liver, and other diseases.
Normal values:
in adults, 1.5-4.5 Bodansky units/dL;
in children, 5.0-14.0 Bodansky units/dL.

Phosphatase, leukocyte alkaline: see Leukocyte alkaline phosphatase test.

Phospholipids: a test done on blood to determine a patient's fat metabolism. *Normal values:* in serum, 6-12 mg/dL (as lipid phosphorous); levels usually somewhat higher in men; pregnant women's levels higher than those of men.

Phosphorus, inorganic: phosphorus measured in the blood as phosphate ions. Elevated levels may indicate kidney, bone, and glandular diseases; lowered levels may indicate alcoholism, vitamin deficiency, and other disease states.
  Normal values: in serum,
      in adults, 1.6-1.8 mEq/L;
      in children, 2.3-4.1 mEq/L.

Phosphorus (in urine): a mineral essential to normal body functioning. Abnormal urine levels may indicate kidney, liver, bone, and other diseases. *Normal values:* in urine after 24-hr collection, 0.9-1.3 g (may vary with intake).

Photometry: see Flame photometry.

Photon absorptiometry: a test done to measure bone density, now done to check for osteoporosis.

Photoscan: a map of the distribution of a radiopharmaceutical in the body.

Phytohemagglutinin test: a test done to detect genetic carriers of cystic fibrosis, an inherited disease that affects the sweat glands and lungs.
  Normal values: in white cells, a noticeable increase in cell protein when exposed to phytohemagglutinin.

Pinocytosis: the process whereby cells take in fluids and change in form.

Pirquet's test: a skin test to detect the presence of, or exposure to, tuberculosis.

Plasma: the fluid portion of blood, including fibrinogen, as distinguished from serum, from which fibrinogen has been separated.

Plasmapheresis: a process in which blood is temporarily withdrawn from a donor via a closed system, the plasma is separated, and the remaining components are returned to the donor. This process is used to obtain blood fractions for patients who need one or more blood components, or to treat disease conditions in the person undergoing plasmapheresis.

Plasma renin activity: the action of renin, an enzyme secreted by the kidney that influences the body's salt and water balance; measured to detect adrenal disease associated with high blood pressure, and to evaluate various predictive factors concerning treatment.
> *Normal values:* in plasma, 0.2-4.0 ng/mL/hr (varies with salt intake and length of time in upright position prior to test).

Plasma volume: measurement of total volume of plasma; elevated in liver and spleen disease and vitamin C deficiency, decreased in dehydration, shock, and Addison's disease.
> *Normal values:* in whole blood,
> in men, 39 mL/kg;
> in women, 40 mL/kg.

Plasminogen: a test done on blood to determine adequacy of the blood clotting process, and to diagnose blood clotting disorders in newborn infants.
> *Normal values:* expressed in percentage of normal, 65% or greater; may also be expressed in activity units, 2.7-4.5 U/mL

Platelet aggregation: a test done on blood to evaluate blood clotting capacity. Excess clotting time indicates a blood clotting deficit, blood disorder, or the presence of drugs that delay normal clotting of blood.
> *Normal values:* clotting is complete in 3-5 min

Platelet count: the number of platelets (thrombocytes) in a sample of whole blood. Platelets, essential in blood clotting, may be reduced in number in some diseases of the blood and after chemotherapy. *Normal values:* 150,000-400,000 per mm^3

Platelet survival: a test done on blood to determine the platelets' length of survival. Low survival rates may indicate certain blood disorders or certain blood- or lymph-borne cancers.
Normal values: the count of radio-labeled platelets is reduced by half within 84-116 hr; all other radioactivity disappears by the end of 8-10 days, considered the normal platelet life span.

Plethysmography: a noninvasive diagnostic technique that measures small changes in the volume of a body part; often used to diagnose abnormal conditions of arteries and veins.

Pleural fluid: the fluid contained in the membranous sac that surrounds each lung.

Pleurisy: inflammation of the double membrane that covers each lung and lines the chest cavity. Pleurisy may cause painful swelling and chafing of the pleural membranes against each other (dry pleurisy) or cause fluid to accumulate between the membranes, compressing the lungs and making breathing difficult (wet pleurisy).

***Pneumocystis carinii* pneumonia:** a form of pneumonia caused by the organism *Pneumocystis carinii* that occurs primarily in people whose immune system is weakened by illness such as AIDS.

Pneumoencephalography: an X-ray study of fluid-containing structures of the brain, using sterile gas injected into the spinal cord as contrast medium.

Pneumonia: inflammation of the lungs, caused by bacteria, viruses, or other organisms, by aspiration of food or fluid, or by the debilitating effects of illness, trauma, or surgery.

Polycystic ovarian disease: a glandular disturbance in some young women. Symptoms involve enlargement of the ovaries with multiple cysts, diminished menstrual flow or absence of periods, excessive hair (hirsutism), and inability to become pregnant.

Polymerase chain reaction: a laboratory technique capable of detecting cells that contain the AIDS (HIV) virus, in its active or inactive form.

Porphobilinogen: a compound present in the urine in porphyria, a congenital metabolic disease.
> *Normal values:* in urine after 24-hr collection,
>> qualitative, negative;
>> quantitative, 0-2.0 mg.

Portable radiography: an X-ray study performed at the patient's bedside with portable X-ray equipment.

Portal hypertension: elevated blood pressure in the liver and nearby blood vessels due to liver disease such as cirrhosis or other conditions that impair circulation through the portal vein.

Positive airway pressure: air flow into the lungs, controlled by a respirator regulating the amount of air and concentration of oxygen delivered to the patient through the respiratory tract or an artificial airway.

Positive end-expiratory pressure: a treatment that provides mechanical breathing assistance for people with respiratory problems that prevent adequate oxygen intake.

Positron emission tomography (PEI): a complex radiologic procedure that assesses biochemical activity in the brain and other organs.

Posterior subcapsular cataract: clouding of the space behind and below the capsule that contains the lens of the eye.

Postherpetic neuralgia: the sensation of pain along certain nerve pathways following a herpesvirus infection.

Postoperative radiography: X-ray studies performed immediately after an operation, in the recovery room, intensive care unit, or patient's room.

Potassium: an essential electrolyte that regulates heart muscle activity, cellular fluid balance, and various enzyme reactions.
Normal values:
in plasma, 3.8-4.5 mEq/L;
in urine after 24-hr collection, 40-80 mEq/L (can vary with diet).

PPD test: see Purified protein derivative test.

Precipitins: antibodies that are capable of reacting with specific soluble antigens to cause precipitation (clumping).

Pregnancy test: see HCG radioreceptor assay.

Pregnanediol: a metabolic product of progesterone; elevated in the urine of women during pregnancy and cyclically with the menstrual cycle; measured to detect ovulation, placental dysfunction, and feminization syndrome in men.
Normal values:
in urine after 24-hr collection,
in men, 0.4-1.4 mg;
in women,
premenopausal, 1-8 mg (peak at one week ovulation)
proliferative phase, 0.5-1.5 mg
leuteal phase, 2.0-7.0 mg
postmenopausal, 0.2-1.0 mg
in children, negative

Pregnanetriol: a progesterone derivative, elevated in adrenogenital disease and Cushing's syndrome.

Normal values: in urine after 24-hr collection,
in men, 1.0-2.0 mg
in women, 0.5-2.0 mg
in children, less than 0.5 mg

Premature atrial beat, atrial premature beat: a skipped heartbeat, flutter sensation, or extra beat. Such beats sometimes occur in people with normal hearts after smoking, drinking coffee, or taking certain drugs. The condition may also occur in people with heart disease.

Premature atrial contraction: see: Premature atrial beat.

Premature ventricular contraction: a skipped heartbeat, also known as extrasystole.

Premenstrual syndrome: a group of symptoms that occur in some women a few days before the onset of their menstrual period. These may include tension, swelling of the breasts, headache, and irritability. Symptoms usually disappear once the period starts.

Preservative: an agent added to fluid (as in food or medicine) that prevents the growth of microbial organisms.

Priapism: a painful, persistent erection not caused by sexual desire but by abnormal circulatory or neurologic condition, or drugs.

Procainamide: a drug used to control irregular or abnormal heart rhythms; monitored to maintain blood levels adequate to control heart rhythm but not high enough to cause toxic reactions.

Therapeutic values: in whole blood drawn 4-6 hr after the most recent dose, 4-8 µg/mL.

Proctitis: inflammation of the mucous membrane of the rectum.

Proctoscopy: direct examination of the anus and rectum with a proctoscope, to detect abnormalities.

Proctosigmoidoscopy: direct examination of the rectum and sigmoid colon with a proctosigmoidoscope, an instrument that penetrates further into the colon than a proctoscope.

Prodrome: symptoms that appear before the actual onset of a disease.

Progesterone test: a test done on blood to determine various reproductive functions, including adequate placental function in a pregnant woman; also tests for causes of infertility and the presence of ovulation.

Progesterone receptor test: a test of a tumor's response to progesterone, to predict whether the tumor is likely to respond to hormonal therapy.

Prolactin (lactogenic hormone): a pituitary hormone that stimulates milk secretion; measured in new mothers with lactation problems, women with menstrual problems, or when brain tumor is suspected.
   Normal values: in serum, 5-25 ng/mL; higher during pregnancy and lactation.

Prophylaxis: treatment or other action intended to prevent the onset of an illness, or to prevent its recurrence if a person has already had it.

Prostate-specific antigen: a substance in blood elevated in patients who have prostate cancer.

Prostatitis: inflammation of the prostate, the male gland that lies just below the urinary bladder, surrounding the urethra (the tube through which urine flows from the bladder during urination).

Protein: a nitrogenous compound found in blood, CSF, and urine, essential to tissue growth and repair. Abnormal blood levels may indicate kidney, liver, and other diseases, abnormal CSF levels may indicate inflammation of the brain or spinal cord or brain hemorrhage; abnormal urine levels may indicate kidney disease.

Normal values:
　　in serum,
　　　　total, 6.0-8.0 g/dL;
　　　　　　albumin, 3.5-5.0 g/dL (52-68% of total);
　　　　　　globulin, 2.0-4.1 g/dL (32-48% of total).
　　in CSF, 15-45 mg/dL (higher, up to 70 mg/dL in elderly and children).
　　in urine after 24-hr collection,
　　　　qualitative, negative;
　　　　quantitative, 10-150 mg.

Protein-bound iodine: iodine chemically bound to protein in the serum; measured as a test of thyroid function.

Normal values: in serum, 4.0-8.0 µg/dL (test results inaccurate if other forms of iodine given previously).

Protein electrophoresis: see Electrophoresis, protein.

Prothrombin consumption test: a test of one of the phases in the blood clotting process; a measure of the blood's ability to generate a normal amount of thromboplastin.

Normal values: in serum, more than 80% of consumption of prothrombin from the serum within 15 sec, or more, measured 1 hr after coagulation.

Prothrombin time (PT): time required for clot formation in plasma; a measure of the activity of several coagulation factors.

Normal values: 12-14 sec

Protoplasm: living matter; the essential substance of which cells are made, composed mainly of nucleic acids, proteins, lipids, carbohydrates, and inorganic salts.

Protoporphyrin: an important natural compound that occurs as an iron complex in hemoglobin and other blood pigments. Elevated levels indicate porphyria (a congenital metabolic disease), lead poisoning, liver disease, or certain cancers.
Normal values: in red blood cells, 27-61 µg/dL packed RBC.

Pruritus: itching.

Psoriasis: a skin disease characterized by itchy red patches covered with dry, silvery scales; noninfectious, but often runs in families.

Pulmonary arteriography: an X-ray study of the pulmonary arteries and related blood vessel structures after injection of contrast medium.

Pulmonary artery wedge pressure: a test that evaluates left heart (atrium) pressure. Done during cardiac catheterization by inserting a thin, plastic catheter into a vein in the arm or neck, advancing it to a central vein (vena cava), and into a vessel in the lung (pulmonary artery).

Purified protein derivative (PPD) test: a skin test done to detect susceptibility or exposure to tuberculosis.

Pus (in feces): a test done to detect infection in the intestinal tract.
Normal values: negative

Pyelography: X-ray studies of the kidneys and urinary tract after injection of contrast medium, to diagnose abnormalities or disease.

Pyelonephritis: an acute or chronic inflammation of the kidneys, usually caused by infection.

Pyruvate: a substance in blood; deficiency causes anemia.
Normal values: in whole blood, 0.3-0.9 mg/dL.

Q

QRS complex: a section of an electrocardiogram tracing that relates to the contraction of the lower heart chambers (ventricles); used in diagnostic studies of the heart.

Quadratic discrimination analysis: a new technique used to screen patients for alcoholism, to test for liver disease, and to distinguish alcoholic liver disease from other types of liver problems. The method consists of applying a specific statistic analysis technique to the results of 25 laboratory tests routinely obtained during hospitalization.

Quality control: a process used in the manufacture of drugs and other medical products that ensures that they meet precise, pre-established standards.

Quantitative radiocardiography: a noninvasive radiologic procedure that measures the flow of blood through the heart and lungs; it can be used as a screening test in healthy patients or for those with heart disease or other conditions.

Quantity not sufficient: terminology used for laboratory specimens submitted in an amount too small to be examined; the report is labeled QNS and returned.

Quantum sufficit: adequate quantity. The term is generally used in the laboratory, to describe a specimen that is of adequate size or quantity to allow examination or analysis.

R

Rabies: a viral disease transmitted to humans by the saliva of an infected animal, often by means of a bite. Immediate treatment and immunization are essential to prevent the virus from traveling via nerve fibers to the brain; if that happens, the infection can cause convulsions, paralysis, and eventually death.

RAD (radiation absorbed dose): a unit of radiation exposure that measures the absorbed dose.

Radarkymography: a noninvasive procedure that shows the size and outline of the heart; electric impulses are passed over the surface of the chest, picked up by radar tracking equipment, and projected on a fluoroscopic screen.

Radiation therapy: treatment by X-rays or other forms of radiation; used to treat cancer and other diseases.

Radioactive decay: the loss of radioactive energy.

Radioactive iodine uptake: a test for thyroid disorders; the thyroid's absorption of oral or intravenous radioactive iodine is measured with a scintillation counter at 1, 6, or 24 hours after ingestion.
> *Normal values:*
>   9-19% in 1 hr
>   7.5-25% in 6 hr
>   10-50% in 24 hr

Radioactivity: the breaking down of atomic nuclei, causing release of alpha, beta, or gamma rays.

Radioallergosorbent assay test: see Radioimmunosorbent assay test.

Radiofrequency (catheter) ablation: a technique in which radio-frequency is used to treat life-threatening irregularities in the heartbeat.

Radiography: the use of X-rays or other forms of radiation to produce an image of a body part.

Radioimmunoassay: a laboratory technique using a radioactive-labeled agent to measure antigens, antibodies, and other proteins in blood plasma.

Radioimmunosorbent assay (RIA): a test using serum immuno-globulin E to detect allergic reactions to environmental substances such as animal hair, grasses, cosmetics, and dust.
   Normal value: in serum, negative.

Radioisotope: an isotope that is radioactive; radioisotopes are used clinically in diagnostic and therapeutic procedures.

Radionuclide: a type of radioactive substance made up of atoms that disintegrate, emitting electromagnetic radiation.

Radiopaque: impenetrable by X-rays or other form of radiation.

Radiopharmaceutical: a radioactive preparation that is injected or given by mouth in certain diagnostic or treatment procedures.

Radiosensitive: capable of being damaged or destroyed by radiation, as a tumor, cell, or tissue.

Range of motion: see: Joint range of motion.

Rapid eye movement (REM): occurs during 20-25% of sleep time, about 5-6 times during the night. It is accompanied by an increased rate and depth of respirations, but depressed muscle tone. REM sleep includes dreaming, and in men, erections occur during the REM sleep cycle.

Rapid plasma reagin test: a blood test to detect syphilis.

Receptors: cellular surface structures that combine with antigens or other substances and thereby acquire new properties.

Recurrent infection: repeat bouts of the same type of infection in the same person.

Red blood cell count: a count of the number of red blood cells in a specimen of whole blood.
> *Normal values:*
> in men, 4.6-6.2 million/mm^3
> in women, 4.2-5.4 million/mm^3

Red blood cell survival time: a test done on blood to find out why a patient has anemia.

Reducing substances, total: a test performed on urine to measure the levels of glucose and other natural sugars.

Refraction (eye): a test done to determine how well a person can see, and whether or what type of correction may be needed, if a vision deficit is found.

Refractive index: a measurement of the total solids in a solution, done by detecting the change in the pathways of light going through the solution.

Remission: a period of time during which there is no evidence of a previously existing disease.

Renal angiography: an X-ray study of the blood vessels surrounding the kidneys, done after injection of contrast medium.

Renal arteriography: an X-ray study of the renal arteries and related blood vessels, done after injection of contrast medium.

Renal scan: a scan of the kidneys for size, shape, and exact location, to diagnose a tumor or other abnormalities; done after intravenous injection of a radioactive substance.

Renin test: see Plasma renin activity.

Resident bacteria: bacteria usually found living in a given body area.

Residual volume: the volume of air that remains in the lungs at the end of maximal expiration.
Normal value: about 1200 mL

Respiratory distress syndrome, acute: a common medical emergency involving respiratory failure due to illness or trauma of the lung; resulting breathing difficulty may become life-threatening unless promptly treated.

Respiratory syncytial virus: a virus that causes acute respiratory illness in children. When infected cells are cultured in a laboratory, a particular clumping of cells becomes apparent and aids in the diagnosis of the infection.

Rest, ice, compression, and elevation (RICE): a combination of methods used to treat injuries of muscles, joints, and surrounding areas that occur during a fall, in sports, or during an accident.

Reticulocyte: a type of red blood cell accounting for about 1% of the red cells in the bloodstream.

Reticulocyte count: a test done to determine the number of reticulocytes in a specimen of whole blood, a measure of bone marrow activity; decreased in hemolytic (blood cell destroying) disease; elevated after hemorrhage, or while recovering from anemia. *Normal values:* 25,000-75,000 mm^3 (0.5-1.5% of red cells).

Retinitis: inflammation of the retina, the innermost part of the eye.

Retrograde pyelogram: a radiographic record of the kidneys and urinary tract, using an instrument inserted in the bladder to inject the contrast medium directly into the urinary tract.

Retrograde urography: see Urography.

Retrolental fibroplasia: a condition in which the posterior portion of the eye's lens develops a fibrous membrane causing near blindness or actual blindness. This condition most often occurs in premature babies who are exposed to large amounts of oxygen while in an incubator during their early days or weeks of life.

Retrovirus: a virus that attacks certain white (T-lymphocyte) blood cells. The AIDS virus is a retrovirus.

Reye's syndrome: an acute, possibly vital disease that occurs most frequently in children. It may follow another illness, such as an upper respiratory infection. Reye's syndrome may begin with vomiting, headache, or sudden change in mental status, which can progress to stupor, coma, and death if not promptly treated. Fatty infiltration of the pancreas, spleen, heart, kidney, lymph nodes, and liver may occur.

Rheumatic fever: an inflammatory disease caused by an untreated streptococcal infection, such as strep throat. Symptoms may include fever, swelling of joints, and nodules under the skin. Heart damage may occur.

Rheumatic heart disease: see: Rheumatic fever.

Rheumatoid arthritis: a disease of unknown cause that produces swelling, inflammation, and pain in various joints, such as those of the fingers, wrists, or toes.

Rheumatoid factor: a blood factor present in rheumatoid arthritis and various other infectious diseases.

Normal values:
    in serum,
        sensitized sheep cell method, a titer of less than 1 : 160;
        latex fixation method, a titer of less than 1 : 80;
        bentonite particles method, a liter of less than 1 : 32.

Rh factor: a blood factor present in most but not all people. An Rh-negative person can develop antibodies to the Rh factor if exposed to it through blood transfusion or pregnancy. An Rh-positive infant of a woman with Rh antibodies may be born with a serious blood disease. Administration of an immune human globulin (RhoGAM) to an Rh-negative mother within 72 hours of giving birth to an Rh-positive infant will prevent the development of antibodies and protect her future pregnancies.

Rh typing: a test done on blood to determine a person's Rh type. Rh-negative women who are married to Rh-positive men require injection of a special product (RhoGAM) to allow normal future pregnancies and delivery of normal babies.

Normal values: Rh-positive, Rh-negative, or Rh-positive D

Ribonucleoprotein: the combination of protein with nucleic acid.

Rickets: a bone disease found primarily in children who don't receive enough vitamin D to allow the proper hardening of bones.

Rickettsiae: tiny microorganisms that live in cells and are considered somewhere between bacteria and viruses in structure.

Right lower quadrant: the lower right portion of the abdomen. This term is used to describe the location of any findings in that area of the abdomen during a physical examination.

Risk reduction: a change in behavior with intent to decrease the likelihood of a specific risk. For example, changing behavior to avoid contracting a sexually transmitted disease.

Roentgen: a unit of measure; the amount of radiation that produces one electrostatic unit of electricity in 1 cubic centimeter of air.

Roentgen equivalent, man: a unit that measures the biologic effect of radiation on the human body.

Rollover test: test done during pregnancy to assess a woman's susceptibility to toxemia of pregnancy, a serious high blood pressure condition of unknown origin.
Normal values: in the pregnant woman, as her position is changed from lying on her left side to lying on her back, no change or elevation of blood pressure is observed.

Rubacell: a blood test done to determine whether a child or adult has had rubella (German measles), to screen for immunity to rubella, and to determine whether a child has congenital rubella infection.

Rubella virus: the virus that causes German measles; see also German measles.

Rubella antibodies: a test done on blood to find out whether a woman is protected against or susceptible to rubella (German measles). Although generally a mild vital disease in children, rubella can cause serious birth defects if contracted by the mother during her first three months of pregnancy.
Normal values: a titer higher than 1 : 10 indicates that the mother is (and her infant will be) protected against the disease.

Rubeola: see measles.

Rule out: a term used in medicine to confirm or exclude a diagnosis. For example, "rule out myocardial infarction" means to diagnose whether the person under examination suffered a heart attack or not.

S

Safe sex: a term used to describe any sexual activity that poses no risk of contracting or transmitting a sexually transmitted disease. Safe sex is only possible if neither partner is infected with a sexually transmitted disease.

Safer sex: a term used to describe any sexual activity that poses a greatly reduced risk of contracting or transmitting a sexually transmitted disease, due to the partners' use of condoms or other devices that make the exchange of infected body fluid unlikely.

Salicylate: a salt of salicylic acid present in blood during treatment with aspirin or aspirin-like drugs.
  Normal value: in serum, negative.
  Therapeutic levels: 150-300 µg/mL.
  Toxic levels: more than 300 µg/mL.

Saliva: fluid secreted by the salivary glands to lubricate the inside of the mouth and help transport and digest food. The usual amount secreted in 24 hours is 1000-1500 mL

Salpingitis: inflammation of a fallopian tube, which carries eggs from the ovary to the uterus.

Saprophyte: an organism that feeds on dead organic matter.

Scabies: an extremely itchy, sexually transmitted infection caused by the mite *Sarcoptes scabiei*, a tiny, insect-like organism related to ticks; causes itchy skin lesions all over the body.

Scarlet fever: a streptococcal disease, once common in childhood, but relatively rare today, probably because of the more common use of antibiotics. The primary symptom is a characteristic rash.

Schick test: a skin test to detect susceptibility or exposure to diphtheria.

Schiller test: a test for abnormalities of the cervix. Iodine is applied to distinguish between normal areas that accept the stain, and abnormal areas, which don't.

Schilling test: a test of vitamin B_{12} blood levels, in which radioactive B_{12} is given orally and measured in 24-hour urine. An abnormal level may be the cause of anemia or other disease conditions. *Normal values:* 8-40% of radioactive B_{12} previously ingested.

Schirmer tearing test: a test done on the eyes to find out if a person is secreting an adequate amount of moisture (tears).
   Normal values: about 10-15 mm of moisture apparent on a paper filter placed in the lower part of the eye.

Schistosomiasis: infection by worms of the genus *Schistosoma*, which penetrate the skin of a person in contact with contaminated water. The worms are carried in the bloodstream to the liver and other parts of the body, causing fever, itching, liver, spleen, and lymph node problems, and a variety of other symptoms, depending on the severity of the infestation. The disease, also known as bilharziasis, affects millions of people in Africa, Asia, South America, and the Caribbean region.

Scintiscan: a map of the distribution in the body, or in a particular body part, of a radioactive compound (radiopharmaceutical) given previously; the emitted rays are printed on photographic film.

Scotch tape swab test: a test done by touching the area surrounding the anus with tape to detect the presence of pinworms, tapeworms, or their eggs.

Scurvy: a disease caused by severe lack of vitamin C. Symptoms include weakness, bleeding gums, and swollen hands and feet.

Secondary infection: a new infection in a person who already has an infection.

Secretin test: a test done to assess pancreatic function by measuring how much pancreatic juice is secreted in response to stimulation by the chemical secretin.

Sedimentation: settling of solid material in blood or other fluid to the bottom of a container.

Sedimentation rate: see Erythrocyte sedimentation rate.

Seizure: see Convulsion.

Seminal fluid, liquefaction: a test of the duration of the liquefaction process in seminal fluid. If delayed, it may indicate abnormalities such as congenital absence of certain internal sexual organs.
Normal value: complete within 20 minutes.

Seminal fluid, morphology: a test of the percentage of normally formed spermatozoa in the seminal fluid; important in fertility studies.
Normal value: more than 70% normal, mature sperm.

Seminal fluid, motility: a test of the percentage of normally motile spermatozoa in the seminal fluid, important in fertility studies.
Normal value: more than 60% of sperm motile.

Seminal fluid, pH: the degree of alkalinity or acidity of seminal fluid, important in fertility studies and diagnostic evaluations of the internal sexual organs.
Normal value: more than 7.0 (average pH is 7.7).

Seminal fluid, sperm count: a test of the quantity of sperm in the seminal fluid; important in fertility studies.
Normal values: 60-150 million sperm/mL (avg: 100 million).

Seminal fluid, volume: a test of the amount of seminal fluid produced during one ejaculation.
Normal values: 1.5-5.0 mL

Senile macular degeneration: deterioration of the macula, a spot on the retina in the rear of the eye near the ocular nerve, which focuses vision. This condition occurs mainly in elderly people, who experience progressively diminishing vision ending in blindness. If diagnosed early enough, macular degeneration can sometimes be arrested with laser treatment.

Sepsis: poisoning of body cells by infectious organisms or by the toxic substances they produce.

Septicemia: poisoning of the bloodstream by infectious organisms or the toxins they produce.

Sequential multiple analysis (SMA-6, SMA-2, SMA-18): the biochemical examination of 6, 12, or 18 blood constituents via a multichannel laboratory apparatus.

Seroconversion: a positive result for an infection in a blood test that at some earlier point in time showed a negative result for the same test.

Serologic test: blood test.

Seronegative: a blood test done for a possible infection that shows a negative result.

Seropositive: a blood test done for a possible infection that shows a positive result.

Serosanguineous fluid: blood and tissue fluids that drain from a wound.

Serotonin: see 5-Hydroxytryptamine.

Seroreverter: a term used to describe a person whose previously positive test for an infection has changed to a negative finding, indicating no infection is currently present. This may occur, for example, in an infant born to an HIV-infected mother, whose antibodies are found in the newborn baby's blood (giving it a positive test result). Once the mother's antibodies disappear from the baby's blood, the baby "seroreverts," i.e. his or her blood (and thus the blood test) becomes negative for HIV antibodies.

Serum: the fluid portion of blood that remains after the blood has clotted.

Serum glutamic-pyruvic transaminase: see Transaminases.

Serum hepatitis: a viral infection of the liver caused by transmission of the virus through a blood transfusion, an intravenous injection, or other access to the blood stream.

Serum sickness: an allergic reaction, usually to an injected drug. May cause fever, joint pains, rash, and swollen lymph glands.

Sex chromatin: a test done on a tissue sample obtained from the membranes that line the inside of the cheek to evaluate the patient for evidence of abnormal sexual development such as ambiguous genitalia, and sexual status in general.

Sexually transmitted disease: any infectious disease that is spread from one person to another by means of sexual contact.

Shingles: see Herpes zoster.

Shock: collapse of the circulatory system, resulting in a dramatic decrease in blood pressure. Symptoms include pale, cold, moist skin; weakness; fast pulse; and shallow breathing. The victim may also be thirsty, nauseous, and void very little urine. Shock may result from trauma, heavy bleeding, severe burns, or illness.

Short of breath: breathlessness or difficulty in breathing resulting from a variety of causes such as strenuous exercise or heart or lung disease.

Sialography: an X-ray study of the parotid and submaxillary glands (situated below and behind the jawbones) after injection of contrast medium.

Sick sinus syndrome: abnormality of the heart's electrical impulse system originating in the upper chambers of the heart (atria).

Sickle cell (hemoglobin-S) test: a test done on blood to determine the presence of sickle-cell disease or sickle-cell trait. (A person with sickle-cell trait who marries another with this trait needs genetic counseling to prevent having a baby with sickle-cell disease.)
Normal value: absence of hemoglobin-S

Sickle-cell disease: a serious, inherited disorder, primarily affecting black people, but which can be found in all races, in which the red blood cells are shaped like sickles. This deformity impairs circulation, leading to anemia, severe joint and abdominal pain, and sometimes stroke, blindness, or kidney disease.

Sigmoidoscopy: internal examination of the sigmoid (lowest portion of the large bowel) with a scope, to detect abnormalities such as a polyp or tumor.

Simian immunodeficiency virus: a virus causing a disease similar to AIDS that occurs in monkeys.

Simplate bleeding time test: a blood test to determine the ability of the platelets to form a plug, the first step in clotting when blood platelets are exposed to air. Delay in forming the plug may be due to platelet deficiency or to a drug such as aspirin.
Normal value: in fresh, standard-size forearm incision, 2-8 min.

Sinus arrhythmia: irregularity of the heartbeat due to a disturbance in an area of the electrical impulse system (sinoatrial node) that controls the heart's actions.

Sinus tachycardia: a rapid heartbeat that may occur following strenuous exercise or as a result of abnormal conditions such as a high fever, hemorrhage, infection, heart disease, and others.

Sleep apnea syndrome: a condition in which a person stops breathing for short periods at intervals while sleeping. This may be due to a respiratory tract abnormality, obesity, heavy snoring, and other causes.

Slit lamp examination: a test done on the eyes to determine possible abnormalities of the anterior eye structures.

SMA: see Sequential multiple analysis.

Smear: a thin layer of tissue or fluid spread on a glass slide for microscopic examination.

Sodium (in blood): a normal blood constituent, essential in transmitting nerve impulses, and in maintaining water metabolism and acid-base balance.
Normal values: in serum, adults, 136-142 mEq/L.

Sodium (in sweat): the level of sodium in sweat, elevated in fibrocystic disease.
Normal values: in sweat, 10-40 mEq/L; (more than 70 mEq/L is indicative of cystic fibrosis).

Sodium (in urine): a normal constituent of urine, measured to check adrenal function, kidney function, acid-base balance, and other conditions.
Normal values: in urine after 24-hr collection, 40-220 mEq/d (depending on diet).

Specific gravity (in urine): the concentration of solutes in a urine specimen compared with a standard specimen; may be altered by disease and other factors.
Normal values: with normal fluid intake, 1.003-1.030.

Specimen: a sample of body tissue or fluid.

Spectrophotometry: see Atomic absorption spectrophotometry.

Speculum: an instrument used to examine the vagina and cervix.

Spinal fluid: see Cerebrospinal fluid.

Spinal tap: to remove fluid from the spinal canal using a needle and syringe.

Spleen scan: a scan of the spleen after injection of radioactive red blood cells, done to detect a tumor, injury, or other abnormality.

Splenoportography: an X-ray study of the spleen, liver, and blood vessels, done after injection of contrast medium into the spleen.

Spore: the reproductive element of fungi and certain bacteria.

Sputum: a mixture of lung and tracheobronchial secretions that are coughed up and may be examined for harmful microorganisms.

Sputum culture: incubation of a sample of sputum in nutrient material to determine the growth and type of infection-causing microorganisms.

ST segment: a section of a tracing taken during an electrocardiogram that provides diagnostic information about the activity of the heart's ventricles.

Stain: a dye that colors bacteria or tissue making them visible to examine under the microscope.

Staphylococcus: a type of disease-causing bacteria that grow in the form of clusters resembling grapes. Common species include *S aureus*, *S epidermidis*, and *S saprophyticus*.

Stereotaxic neuroradiography: an X-ray procedure, generally done in the operating room during neurosurgery, helpful in guiding the insertion of a needle into a desired location in the brain.

Sterile: free of microorganisms.

Steroid hormones: the sex hormones and adrenal cortical hormones.

Still's disease: see Juvenile rheumatoid arthritis.

Stomatitis: inflammatory condition of the mouth that may be due to a variety of causes including vitamin deficiency, allergy, infection, and trauma.

Stool culture: incubation of a sample of feces in nutrient material to determine growth and types of infection-causing microorganisms.

Strangulated hernia: a condition in which an organ protruding through a weakened area of tissue is cut off from its blood supply.

Streptococcal MG agglutinin test: a test for pneumonia or other pulmonary infections caused by certain streptococcus strains.
Normal values: in serum, a titer of less than 1 : 20.

Streptococcus: a type of disease-causing bacteria that grow in the form of chains. Common species include *S pneumoniae* and *S pyogenes*.

Streptolysins O and S: the poisonous substances produced by certain forms of streptococci; known as beta hemolytic because they can destroy blood cells.

Stress electrocardiogram: an ECG tracing made while the patient exercises on a treadmill or stationary bicycle, to evaluate heart muscle function.
Normal value: while exercising, no change in ECG, except for an increase in heart rate.

Stress test: see Exercise electrocardiography.

String test: see Entero test.

Stroke: see Cerebrovascular accident.

Subacute bacterial endocarditis: infection of the valves or the membrane that lines the heart, caused by a streptococcal organism that lives in these areas. This condition usually occurs in a person with a damaged heart due to an illness such as rheumatic fever.

Subdural hemorrhage: bleeding into the space between the dura mater and the arachnoid membranes that cover the brain; due to injury or illness.

Sudden unexplained death: death that occurs unexpectedly in a previously healthy person, who had given no indication that sudden death was likely to occur.

Sudden infant death syndrome (SIDS): sudden, unexpected death of an infant or very small child. May be due to a previously unrecognized infection, allergy, respiratory illness, or as yet unknown causes. Some research points to infant sleeping position.

Sulfhemoglobin: a substance not normally present in the blood, but found in patients who have taken an excess of certain drugs, or in cases of hydrogen sulfide poisoning.

Sulfobromophthalein: chemical used in liver function tests. Injected intravenously, its retention in the blood is measured after a period of time. *Normal value:* less than 6% retained after 45 min.

Sulfonamides: a class of bacteriostatic medications used to treat infection.

Superinfection: growth of certain harmful organisms normally kept in check by other organisms that are temporarily destroyed by an antibiotic medication.

Surgical sponge radiography: an X-ray study done to locate a surgical sponge in the operative area during, or just after, surgery.

Surrogate markers: examination of certain cells or blood proteins that indirectly indicate activity of the AIDS virus (HIV).

Susceptibility: the state of being receptive to infection or disease.

Sweat test: measurement of sodium and chloride concentrations in sweat to diagnose cystic fibrosis. Very high levels indicate the disease is present.
   Normal values:
      sodium, 10-40 mmol/L (more than 70 mmol/L is indicative of cystic fibrosis);
      chloride, 0-30 mmol/L (60-200 mmol/L is indicative of cystic fibrosis).

Syncope: fainting.

Syndrome: a set of symptoms that tend to appear together.

Synovial fluid: viscid fluid secreted by the membrane that lines a joint cavity.

Synovial fluid-blood glucose difference: the difference in glucose levels between blood and synovial fluid, which may be increased in arthritis and certain other conditions.
   Normal difference: less than 10 mg/dL

Synovial fluid, differential cell count: a test in which cells are differentiated and counted to detect inflammation or infection.
Normal values: granulocytes constitute fewer than 25% of nucleated cells.

Synovial fluid, fibrin clot: a clot present during inflammation or infection.

Synovial fluid, mucin clot: a clot whose quality may be fair to poor in inflammation or infection.
Normal value: firm

Synovial fluid, nucleated cell count: a count elevated in inflammatory or infectious conditions, as well as after hemorrhage.
Normal values: fewer than 200 cells/μL

Synovial fluid, viscosity: a property that may be decreased in inflammatory or septic conditions.
Normal value: high

Synovial fluid, volume: the amount of synovial fluid in a joint, which may be increased in trauma or other abnormal conditions.
Normal values: less than 3.5 mL

Syphilis: a sexually transmitted disease caused by a bacterium called *Treponema pallidum.* The disease may be cured if treated with antibiotics as soon as it first occurs. Untreated syphilis may lead to severe cardiovascular or neurologic complications and, if present in a pregnant woman, may cause congenital syphilis in the baby.

Systemic lupus erythematosus: see: Lupus erythematosus.

Systole: the portion of the heart cycle during which its chambers contract.

T

T and B lymphocyte assay: a test done on blood to determine whether a patient has any immunodeficiency disease, or other white blood cell disease that produces an excess of lymphocytes (a type of white blood cell).
Normal values:
  T cells, 68-75% of total lymphocytes
  B cells, 10-20% of total lymphocytes
  total lymphocyte count, 1500-3000/mm^3
    T cell count, 1400-2700/mm^3
    B cell count, 64-475/mm^3

T cell: a white blood cell that defends the body by killing foreign cells.

T-cell mediated immunity: immunity against certain infections, allergies, and other diseases whose effectiveness is based on the number of T-cells present in blood.

T-helper (CD4) cell: a white blood cell (lymphocyte) that helps to protect the body against foreign materials or organisms.

T-helper/T-suppressor ratio: a ratio between two different types of white blood cells that, when normal, preserves the body's immune status and so helps it to fight infection. The ratio is tested to determine a person's immune status (competence). It is often performed on patients who are HIV-infected or have AIDS.
Normal values: T4/T8 ratio, 1-3.5

T-suppressor cell: a white blood cell (lymphocyte) released when foreign substances such as an infectious organism invade the body.

T wave: a section of an electrocardiogram tracing that indicates the lower heart chambers (ventricles) are ready to fill with blood; used in diagnostic studies of the heart.

Tachycardia: an abnormally rapid heartbeat.

Tachypnea: abnormally rapid respirations.

Tangent-screen examination: a test done on the eyes to detect visual field loss or increase or decrease in visual field loss.
Normal value: no loss of vision throughout the visual field.

Tartrazine sensitivity: sensitivity to tartrazine, a substance found in some foods (eg, sweet potatoes) and used as a color additive in foods and drugs.

Tay-Sachs disease: a progressive disease in infants that involves deterioration of the brain and results in death at an early age.

Technetium-pyrophosphate scanning: a test done to determine whether and to what extent heart muscle has been damaged after a heart attack. The test is done by injecting intravenously first a tracer isotope, and, several hours later, a radioactive chemical. A scintillation camera or scanner is then used to take multiple images of the heart. The results indicate whether and to what extent the patient's heart muscle is damaged.

Temperature, pulse, respirations: these vital signs are taken during a physical examination, and during an illness as a basic, important evaluation of a patient's condition.

Temporomandibular joint dysfunction: pain in the region of the lower jawbone (mandible) and the temporal bone situated in front of the ear.

Terminal deoxynucleotidyl transferase (TdT): a test done on blood or bone marrow to detect certain types of leukemia or lymphoma. For bone marrow cells, bone marrow aspiration must be done from the breast bone or the hip. *Normal values:* TdT levels 0-10 IU/10^{13} cells

Terminal disinfection: a method of removing disease-causing organisms and their toxins from a room previously occupied by a patient who had an infectious disease.

Terminal infection: an infection that causes death.

Test of diffusing capacity (DLCO): measurement of the way in which carbon monoxide diffuses (moves) across the alveocapillary-erythrocyte membrane in the lung. Carbon monoxide is used because it is similar to oxygen, but easier to measure.
Normal values: 25-35 mL/min/mm Hg

Test of distribution of inspired air: a test done to measure the change in nitrogen concentration at the peak of exhalation after the patient takes a deep breath of oxygen.
Normal values: in alveolar gases, less than 2% change in nitrogen concentration between 750 mL and 1250 mL of the exhalation.

Test of perfusion: a test done to measure the ratio of ventilation to perfusion (blood flow through the capillaries) in the lung.
Normal values: after breathing 100% oxygen for 10-20 min, a five-fold increase or more in arterial oxygen pressure (PO$_2$).

Testosterone: a male sex hormone present in blood; important in diagnosing poor function of the testes (decreased level) and testicular cancer (increased level).
Normal values: in serum or plasma,
in men, 275-875 ng/dL;
in women, 23-75 ng/dL (38-190 ng/dL in pregnant women).

Tetanus: a serious infection caused by a *Clostridium* bacterium, causing severe muscle spasm, including clamping of the jaw (lockjaw). Acquired through puncture or other wounds. Immunization prevents the infection.

Tetany: muscle cramps, spasms, and sometimes convulsions associated with low blood levels of calcium.

Tetralogy of Fallot: a combination of deformities found in some newborn infants, consisting of defects in the heart's walls and blood vessels. Surgery can often correct this condition.

Thallium 201 stress test: a procedure in which an isotope of the metal Thallium is injected into the vein of a person who has been doing prescribed, measured exercises for some time. A gamma-scintillation camera is then used to take images of the heart muscle to check blood flow. A smaller than usual uptake of Thallium 201 in any area indicates a decreased blood flow in that area. The test is repeated after a rest of several hours. Blood flow at that time may still be decreased, indicating some abnormality, or it may be adequate, indicating that blood flow is adequate for non-stressful activities, but not sufficient during exertion.

Thallium imaging: a test done to determine how much blood is able to circulate through the heart muscle. The test is done by injecting a radioactive substance intravenously, followed by producing images of the heart with a scintillation camera or a scanner. Other heart-related tests (electrocardiogram, blood pressure measurements) are taken while the patient works out on a treadmill or a stationary bicycle.

Therapeutic abortion: an abortion that may be performed if the mother is at risk of serious physical or mental harm should her pregnancy continue, if the fetus is found to have serious abnormalities, or if rape is the cause of the pregnancy.

Therapeutic drug monitoring: monitoring of drug blood levels during treatment to achieve maximum therapeutic effect and minimal toxicity.

Thermography: measurement of temperature variations in soft tissues; a useful technique for detecting various abnormalities.

Thoracentesis: removal of fluid from inside the chest wall with a syringe and needle, for diagnosis or treatment purposes.

Throat culture: incubation of a sample of throat secretions in nutrient material, to determine the presence and type of infection-causing microorganisms.

Thrombin: a chemical substance in blood that causes it to begin to clot once it is no longer inside the body. See Bleeding and clotting time.

Thrombin time: see: Bleeding and clotting time.

Thromboangiitis obliterans: a chronic disease of the blood vessels that occurs mainly in the smaller (peripheral) arteries and veins. Symptoms include periodic flare-ups of inflammation and blood clots in the affected blood vessels.

Thrombocytopenic purpura: a blood disease whose symptoms include periodic hemorrhages into the skin, a defective clotting mechanism, and deficiency of blood platelets. Removal of the spleen often cures this condition.

Thrombophlebitis: formation of a blood clot in a vein, most often in the leg, accompanied by inflammation; may also occur at site of intravenous line.

Thrombosis: a blood clot, usually in the heart or in a blood vessel.

Thromboplastin generation time: the time it takes whole blood to generate thromboplastin, a coagulation factor. Deficient thromboplastin generation causes bleeding problems.
Normal values: 12 sec or less (100%)

Thrush: an infection of the mucous membranes of the mouth caused by a fungus, usually *Candida albicans*. Also known as moniliasis.

Thymol flocculation (turbidity): a test to determine the functional capacity of the liver, performed by mixing a serum sample with thymol. Increased turbidity (cloudiness) indicates liver disease such as hepatitis. *Normal values:* in serum, 0-5 turbidity units.

Thyroid antibodies: antibodies present in various diseases, such as autoimmune thyroid disease, allergic disorders, and pernicious anemia.
Normal values: in serum,
    antithyroglobulin antibody, a titer of less than 1:32;
    antithyroid microsomal antibody, a titer of less than 1:56.

Thyroid hormone tests: (triiodothyronine, T_3; thyroxine, T_4; thyroxine-binding globulin, TBG): tests done to determine the levels of thyroid hormones for diagnosing various thyroid disorders.
Normal values: in serum:
    expressed as iodine,
        T_4 (by column), 3.2-7.2 µg/dL
        T_4 (by competitive binding), 3.9-7.7 µg/dL
        free T_4, 0.6-3.3 ng/dL
    expressed as thyroxine,
        T_4 (by column), 5-12 µg/dL
        T_4 (by competitive binding), 6-11.8 µg/dL
        free T_4, 1.0-2.1 ng/dL
        T_3 (resin uptake), 25-38% relative uptake
        TBG, 10-26 µg/dL

Thyroid scan: an imaging procedure done after injecting a radioactive substance into a vein, to determine the thyroid's size, shape, location, and function, or any abnormality such as cancer.

Thyroid-stimulating immunoglobulin test: a blood test done to determine the presence of thyroid-stimulating immunoglobulins, indicative of thyroid disease.

Thyroid stimulation test: a procedure in which the patient is given thyroid-stimulating hormone (TSH), a secretion of the pituitary gland. Its effects on the thyroid are then observed to determine whether thyroid problems are due to pituitary or thyroid dysfunction.

Thyroid-131 uptake: a test for thyroid disorders; the thyroid's absorption of oral or intravenous radioactive iodine is measured with a scintillation counter at 1, 6, or 24 hours after ingestion.
Normal values:
   9-19% in 1 hr
   7.5-25% in 6 hr
   10-50% in 24 hr

Thyroxine: a thyroid hormone measured in venous blood; elevated in hyperthyroidism and decreased in hypothyroidism. See Thyroid hormone tests.

Thyroxine binding globulin: if elevated, indicates various disease states and metabolic abnormalities. If levels are low, hyperthyroidism, malnutrition, kidney disease and various other disease conditions may be the cause. See Thyroid hormone tests.

Tidal volume: the amount (volume) of gas inhaled or exhaled during a respiratory cycle. *Normal value:* about 500 mL.

Timed forced expiratory volume: a measurement of lung capacity. *Normal values:* 80% air exhaled in first sec and 95% air exhaled by the third sec.

Tinnitus: ringing in the ears due to a variety of causes, such as a disorder of the ear.

Tissue: an accumulation of cells that forms an identifiable structure, such as skin.

Tissue culture: the process of growing cells outside the body for various diagnostic or research purposes.

Titer: the strength, or concentration, of a substance in fluid, such as the lowest dilution of serum at which antibody is still present.

Tomography: a special X-ray technique that visualizes layers of tissues.

Tonometry: the use of an instrument (tonometer) to measure the fluid pressure inside the eyeball, mainly to test for glaucoma, a condition in which fluid pressure is elevated.

Topfer's test: a test for free hydrochloric acid in the stomach. Done by adding 1 or 2 drops of a solution (Topfer's reagent) to 5 drops of gastric juice.
  Normal value: cherry red color if free gastric acid is present

Total body irradiation: a process which subjects the entire body to irradiation, used in the treatment of certain cancers or to eliminate rejection of a transplanted organ or tissues.

Total hip replacement: a surgical procedure in which a damaged or diseased hip joint is replaced by a mechanical device that works like the original hip joint, allowing improved hip joint mobility.

Total iron-binding capacity: see Iron-binding capacity.

Total lung capacity: see Total lung volume.

Total lung volume: the size of the lungs and their space, in liters, measured by having the patient rebreathe a gas such as helium.

Tourniquet test: a test done to check for the presence of certain blood diseases, or for scurvy.
Normal values: after placement of a tourniquet (blood pressure cuff) inflated for up to 15 min, no new hemorrhagic spots (petechiae).

Toxemia: a condition in which toxins produced by bacteria poison the bloodstream, usually as a result of an overwhelming infection.

Toxic shock syndrome: a severe, sometimes life-threatening infection that may occur when highly absorbent menstrual tampons are kept in the vagina for an unusually long period of time. Researchers believe that such conditions allow the development of a toxin produced by the Staphylococcus aureus organism, which causes symptoms such as high fever, chills, diarrhea, weakness, and low blood pressure. Occasionally diagnosed in men.

Toxin: a poisonous metabolic product of a living organism, usually of disease-causing microorganisms such as bacteria.

Toxoid: a product prepared from bacterial toxins that has been treated so it is no longer toxic but can still stimulate the production of antitoxin against bacterial infections such as diphtheria or tetanus. It is therefore a useful agent in immunization.

Toxoplasma antibodies: antibodies to the parasite *Toxoplasma gondii*, which causes toxoplasmosis, an infectious disease often spread via cat feces. *Normal values:* in serum, a titer of less than 1 : 4.

Toxoplasmosis: an infection caused by the organism *Toxoplasma gondii*, which may be found in cat feces and can be transmitted to humans. May develop as an opportunistic infection in AIDS or HIV-infected patients.

Transaminases: the enzymes serum glutamic-oxaloacetic transaminase (SGOT), also known as aspartate aminotransferase, and serum glutamic-pyruvic transaminase (SGPT), also known as alanine amino-transferase. Blood levels of these enzymes are measured to diagnose liver and heart disease.
Normal values:
in serum:
SGOT, 7-40 U/L (37oC)
SGPT, 5-35 U/L (37oC)

Transferrin: an iron-binding protein in the blood; levels are increased in iron deficiency and decreased in inflammatory conditions and liver disease.
Normal values: in serum, 220-400 mg/dL.

Transfusion: the injection of fluid, blood, or blood components into a vein to counteract depletion of fluid, blood, or blood components.

Transfusion-associated AIDS: AIDS contracted via a transfusion with AIDS-contaminated blood.

Transient ischemic attack: a sudden neurologic disturbance due to a temporary lack of adequate blood supply caused by cerebral artery spasm. May cause brief periods of inability to move or speak. Recurrent attacks may be predictive of stroke.

Transrectal ultrasonography: an ultrasound procedure done to diagnose cancer of the prostate.

Treadmill stress test: a test to assess fitness and possible abnormalities of the cardiovascular system. An electrocardiogram is done while the patient is exercising; the test is stopped if an abnormality is noted.

Trench mouth: see:Necrotizing ulcerative gingivitis.

Treponema pallidum: the organism that causes syphilis.

Trichina (Trichinella) agglutinin test: a test performed to detect the presence of trichinosis, a disease contracted by persons who eat undercooked, infected pork or beef.

Trichinosis: an illness caused by a parasitic roundworm, *Trichinella spiralis*, that is transmitted to humans by eating undercooked beef or pork. Early symptoms include nausea, vomiting, fever, diarrhea, and abdominal pain. Once the larvae move from the digestive tract to other body areas, muscle pain and inflammation develop, with fever, edema of the eyelids, and sometimes severe respiratory, neurologic, and cardiac symptoms.

Trichomonas wet preparation: a test done on penile discharge (in men) and on cervical mucus (in women) to detect the presence of the sexually transmitted disease trichomoniasis, which is caused by the protozoa *Trichomonas vaginalis*. A sample of the secretions is examined either immediately under a microscope, or cultured.
Normal value: no trichomonads seen

Trichomoniasis: a sexually transmitted disease (infection) caused by the protozoa *Trichomonas vaginalis*, which may cause a variety of genital symptoms. It may also be present without any symptoms.

Triglycerides: fatty substances measured in the blood. They may be elevated in the presence of heart and blood vessel diseases.
Normal values: in serum, fasting, 40-150 mg/dL

Triiodothyronine (T_3) resin uptake: incorporation of radioactive T_3 and synthetic resin particles by serum, tested to determine whether the patient has hyperthyroidism or hypothyroidism.

Trypsin activity test: a test done on feces for the presence of trypsin; done to diagnose fibrocystic disease of the pancreas, respiratory system, sweat glands, or other organ systems.
Normal values: in random, fresh feces, trypsin 2+ to 4+.

Tuberculin: a substance derived from tubercle bacilli (tuberculosis-causing organisms), used to diagnose tuberculosis or exposure to the disease.

Tuberculin test: a skin test using tuberculin to detect susceptibility or exposure to tuberculosis. *Normal value:* no reaction

Tuberculosis: an infectious disease caused by the organism *Mycobacterium tuberculosis.* It generally attacks the lungs, but may also affect other organs, such as the stomach, lymph nodes, or bones. The disease is transmitted primarily by inhalation of droplets emitted by an infected person. It is treated with drugs.

Tubo-ovarian abscess: a pus-filled area in the fallopian tube and the ovary. This may occur in women who have pelvic inflammatory disease (one or more sexually transmitted diseases that travel through the genital tract). This condition causes intense pain in the abdominal area, requiring surgical treatment.

Tularemia agglutinin test: a test done to determine the presence of tularemia, an infectious disease spread through contact with infected rabbits.
Normal values: in serum, a titer of less than 1 : 80.

Tumor doubling time: the length of time it takes a cancerous cell mass to double in bulk (cell mass). These measurements are important in calculating cancer therapy.

Tumor necrosis factor: a substance released by certain malignant tumors.

Tuning-fork tests: tests in which a tuning fork is used to measure hearing function and bone-conduction sensitivity in various neurologic (nervous system) examinations.

Turbidimetry: measurement of the transmission of light through a suspension, used to determine the presence of protein in urine, spinal fluid, or plasma, and in the quantitative determination of bacteria and antigen-antibody complexes.

Tympanometry: a test done to determine whether allergy or infection is interfering with adequate functioning of the eardrum. Varying tones are administered to the outer ear canal, and the pressure response within the ear is recorded on a graph.

Typhoid agglutinin test: a test done on serum to diagnose the presence of typhoid fever.
Normal values:
    O, a titer below 1 : 80
    H, a titer below 1 : 80

Type and crossmatch: a blood test done before a blood transfusion is administered. The donor's blood as well as the recipient's blood is tested to be sure both are of the same blood type; donor and recipient blood samples are then mixed to confirm that their bloods are compatible, and will not clot when the transfusion is given.

Typing: classifying blood, tissues, cells, disease-causing organisms, and other materials so they can be compared with standards.

U

Ulcer: an opening in the skin or mucous membrane that has become sore and inflamed. May occur outside or inside the body.

Ulcerative colitis: a chronic disease of unknown cause. It affects portions of the colon or rectum, producing ulcers, bleeding, and other complications in these areas.

Ultrasound: high-frequency sound waves used to project images of various parts of the body. A transducer applied to the skin produces the ultrasound and catches the response, which is displayed on an oscilloscope. Often used to assess fetal development at various stages of pregnancy.

Ultrasonography: the measurement of interior body structures by means of ultrasonic waves, with special computerized equipment that can translate the reflection of the sound waves into images.

Unknown origin: a term used to describe a medical fact, symptom, or illness whose cause has not been determined.

Unsaturated vitamin B_{12} binding capacity: a test that measures the ability of vitamin B_{12} to bind with a protein called intrinsic factor in the stomach, prior to absorption in the bowel.
Normal values: in serum, 1-2 ng/mL of free vitamin B_{12}.

Upper respiratory tract infection: infection involving the nose, paranasal passages, throat, larynx, trachea, and bronchi.

Urea clearance: the amount of urea filtered and removed from the blood by the kidneys within a given period of time.
Normal values: in serum and urine, maximum clearance, 64-99 mL/min; standard clearance, 41-65 mL/min, or more than 75% of normal clearance.

Urea nitrogen: a nitrogen fraction elevated in the serum and urine of patients with certain kidney and other diseases.
> *Normal values:*
>> in serum, 11-23 mg/dL;
>> in urine after 24-hr collection, 6-17 g.

Uremia: a generalized toxic condition caused by the failure of the kidneys to eliminate waste materials. Symptoms include vomiting, headache, dizziness, an odor of urine on the breath, poor vision, and seizures. Uremia may be caused by acute or chronic illness of the kidneys, overwhelming infection, and by trauma such as burns or shock. Treatment: Hemodialysis.

Urethritis: inflammation of the urethra, the urinary canal leading from the urinary bladder to the external opening, which discharges the urine.

Uric acid: a substance elevated in the serum and urine in various diseases such as gout, and decreased if the patient is taking anticoagulants or antiworm medication.
> *Normal values:*
>> in serum,
>>> in men, 3.5-7.2 mg/dL
>>> in women, 2.6-6.0 mg/dL
>> in urine, 250-750 mg/24 hr

Urinary creatinine clearance: see Creatinine.

Urinary tract infection: infection involving the urethra, urinary bladder, ureters, or kidneys.

Urine protein electrophoresis: a laboratory procedure that uses electrical potential to move colloidal particles (urinary proteins) through the solution in which they are disbursed. The different proteins and protein mixtures present are analyzed by measuring the speed at which they move.

Urine specimen, 24-hour: all the urine voided in a 24-hour period; necessary for certain urine tests, such as the creatinine clearance test.

Urobilinogen, (urinary): a bilirubin metabolism product found in urine and stool; a test is done to aid in the diagnosis of liver disease, bile-duct disease, to evaluate how well the liver and bile ducts function, and to detect disorders of red blood cells.
> *Normal values:* up to 1.0 Ehrlich unit/2 hr (1-3 p.m.), or 0.0-4.0 mg/ 24 hr.

Urodynamics: diagnostic procedures that measure changes in pressure inside the bladder with volume over time.

Uroflowmetry: a test done with special equipment while patient urinates that helps determine how well the urinary tract is functioning, and whether there is an obstruction at the outlet of the bladder.
> *Normal values:* variable, since urine flow rate varies depending on a person's sex, age, and volume of urine voided

Urography: an X-ray procedure used to diagnose abnormalities of the genitourinary tract. Intravenous urography involves intravenous injection of a contrast medium that allows visualization of the blood vessels of the kidneys and ureters. Retrograde urography involves visualization of the urinary tract by cystoscopy, bladder catheterization, and infusion of radiopaque material through the catheter.

Uroporphyrins: substances present in the urine in congenital or metabolic disease, such as porphyria.
> *Normal values:*
> qualitative, random specimen, absent;
> quantitative, 24-hr specimen, 10-30.

V

Vaccination: introduction of an antibody-stimulating substance (antigen) into the body.

Vaccine: a substance made from disease-causing material that has been modified so it will not cause disease when introduced into the body but will stimulate the formation of antibodies to that disease.

Vaginal dryness: a common complaint in older women, especially following menopause. The vaginal lining becomes dry and may crack and/or bleed, resulting in painful intercourse. Cause: Reduced levels of female hormone (estrogen). This condition can be greatly improved by using a vaginal moisturizer from any pharmacy. A doctor may prescribe estrogen in the form of a vaginal cream, pills, or a patch to restore the damaged vaginal lining to a healthy condition.

Vaginitis: inflammation of the tissues of the vagina.

Valsalva maneuver: forceful breathing out (exhaling) to open a clogged auditory (ear) tube, or to modify certain heart irregularities.

Vanillylmandelic acid: see 3-Methoxy-4-hydroxymandelic acid.

Varicella-zoster virus: the virus that causes shingles, also known as herpes zoster. See Herpes zoster.

Varicose veins: twisted, often enlarged veins in the legs and other body areas such as the rectum, the vagina, and the esophagus. Causes may be occupational, such as a job that requires standing for long periods, as well as obesity, pregnancy, constipation, and liver disease. Treatment depends on the location and severity of the varicose veins.

Vasectomy: surgical removal of a portion of a man's vas deferens (spermatic duct), usually performed to induce sterility.

Vasopressin concentration test: a test that measures the ability of urine to concentrate; used to diagnose certain diseases in which urine has a low level of concentration (specific gravity).
Normal values: in urine after subcutaneous injection of 10 UPS units of vasopressin, specific gravity of more than 1.020 in urine collected after 60 and 120 min.

Vector: a carrier of disease-causing microorganisms from one host to another (eg, a fly, louse, or mosquito).

Vectorcardiogram, spatial: a three-dimensional electrocardiogram that shows electric activity in the heart muscle projected on three coordinates simultaneously, as well as muscle contraction and relaxation.

Vein scan: a scanning procedure performed after intravenous injection of a radiopharmaceutical, to detect blood clots or inflammation.

Venereal: caused or spread by sexual contact.

Venereal Disease Research Laboratory test: a blood test for syphilis.
Normal values: in serum, nonreactive.

Venography: a radiographic procedure that shows the internal structures of veins after the patient receives an injection of contrast medium.

Venous impedance plethysmography: a procedure that measures blood flow through a vein to detect the presence of a clot.

Venous thrombosis: a blood clot in a vein.

Ventilation scan (lung scan): a procedure in which the patient breathes in radioactive gas and the lungs are scanned for areas that don't receive air, or other abnormalities.

Ventricular fibrillation: grossly abnormal heartbeat, sometimes described as a quivering motion, that causes death if not treated immediately. Usually caused by a serious abnormality in the electrical impulse system that governs the heart's cycle of activity. When this condition is present, electrical impulses in the upper chambers of the heart occur continuously, throw off the heart's regular rhythm, and cause a very fast pulse rate, palpitations, feelings of fainting, nausea, weakness, and fatigue. Treatment: Drug therapy to slow down the beat. Cardioversion, a procedure that shocks the heart back into a regular rhythm, may also be used.

Ventricular gallop: an abnormal heart sound heard in a person with serious heart disease and a rapid heartbeat of 100 or more per minute.

Ventricular tachycardia: excessively rapid heartbeat (arrhythmia) originating in the ventricle, which causes low blood pressure, shock, build-up of fluid in the lungs, and sometimes, palpitations. This condition occurs primarily in people who have serious heart disease, and must be treated as an emergency. Several drugs are used to treat this problem. Cardioversion is employed to stabilize the heart's rhythm if ventricular tachycardia follows a heart attack.

Ventriculography: an X-ray study of the ventricles of the brain, involving the insertion of needles to withdraw fluid and inject air or gas.

Very-low-density lipoprotein cholesterol: a cholesterol fraction which, when elevated, may predispose to hardening of the arteries and heart disease.

Vertigo: dizziness.

Vincent's disease: see: Acute necrotizing ulcerative gingivitis.

Viral hepatitis: see: Hepatitis.

Viral respiratory infection: an infection of the breathing passages caused by a virus.

Viremia: a vital infection of the blood.

Virulence: the capacity of a given organism or group of organisms to produce disease of various degrees of severity.

Virus: a tiny particle of protein and nucleic acid that is able to pass into living cells and cause changes in the chemistry of the cell. Many viruses are capable of causing disease.

Virus-neutralizing antibodies: antibodies that render a virus harmless.

Viscosity: glue-like or sticky property of a semi-liquid substance. *Normal values:* in whole blood, 1.4-1.8 times that of water.

Visual acuity tests: tests done on the eyes to determine whether a person is near or farsighted.
Normal values:
distance acuity, 20/20 (the patient can read letters of 6 cm size at a distance of 20 feet);
near acuity, 14/14 (a person can read letters or other visual symbols at a distance of 14 feet).

Visual evoked potential: use of a series of stimuli during an electroencephalogram (EEG) to determine, with the help of computer averaging, any optic nerve deficiency in patients with multiple sclerosis.

Visual field: the area visible to the eye.

Vital capacity: lung volume; measured as the patient breathes in, then exhales as much air as possible.
Normal values: about 4-6 L/exhalation

Vital signs: indications of a person's health status that include the pulse and respiratory rate, blood pressure, and temperature.

Vitamin A (retinol): a fat-soluble vitamin present in inadequate amounts in poor nutrition and in certain other conditions, such as with use of oral contraceptives or excessive consumption of mineral oil.
Normal values: in serum, 20-80 µg/dL.

Vitamin A tolerance: a test of the body's capacity to react to a given dose of vitamin A. Failure of serum levels to rise to normal within 4-5 hours indicates inadequate intestinal fat absorption.
Normal values:
    in serum (after giving 5000 U vitamin A/kg in oil),
        fasting, 15-60 µg/dL after;
        3 to 6 hours, 200-600 µg/dL;
        after 24 hr, fasting level or slightly higher.

Vitamin B₁ (thiamine): a vitamin present in inadequate amounts in poor nutrition, alcoholism, and other conditions.
Normal values:
    in whole blood, 1.5-4.0 µg/dL;
    in urine, 25-75 µg/dL.

Vitamin B₂ (riboflavin): a vitamin whose deficiency may cause eye and skin problems as well as abnormal states of the blood and nervous system.
Normal values:
    in blood, over 15 µg/dL of red blood cells;
    in 6-hr urine collection, 0.6-1.5 µg.

Vitamin B₃ (niacin): a vitamin whose deficiency may cause skin, nervous system, and intestinal problems. Deficiency may be caused by alcoholism.
Normal values: in 6-hr urine collection, 0.6-1.5 mg.

Vitamin B₆ (pyridoxine): a vitamin whose deficiency may cause eye, skin, mouth, and nervous system problems.
Normal values: in urine after 24-hr collection, 35-55 µg.

Vitamin B₁₂ (cyanocobalamin) test: a test of the body's ability to absorb and utilize vitamin B₁₂; decreased in pernicious anemia, after surgical removal of the stomach, in alcoholism, gastrointestinal infection, and various other conditions.
Normal values:
in serum,
in men, 200-800 pg/mL;
in women, 100-650 pg/mL.
in urine, 8-40% of the radioactive vitamin B₁₂ previously ingested by mouth.

Vitamin C (ascorbic acid): a vitamin whose deficiency may cause skin, gum, and hair problems, and interfere with tooth and bone development.
Normal values:
in plasma, 0.6-2.0 mg/dL;
in urine after 24-hr collection, more than 50 mg.

Vitamin D, alkaline phosphatase test: a test to detect vitamin D deficiency, which may cause rickets, softening of the bones (osteomalacia), muscle weakness, and tooth decay.
Normal values: in serum,
in adults, 2.0-4.5 Bodansky units/dL;
in children, 5-15 Bodansky units/dL.

Vitamin E (tocopherol): a vitamin whose deficiency may cause anemia and infertility.
Normal values: in serum, 7-20 µg/mL.

Vitamin K: a vitamin whose deficiency may cause inadequate clotting of the blood.

Normal values: in plasma, 12-14 see (prothrombin time).

Vollmer test: a patch (skin) test to determine the presence of tuberculosis or previous exposure to the disease.

Volume, total: the total amount of urine excreted in a 24-hour period; measured to assess kidney function. *Normal values:* 600-1600 mL/24 hr.

Vulvitis: inflammation of the external female genitalia.

W

Wasting syndrome: a group of symptoms that may develop in an HIV-infected person with AIDS-related complex before developing full-blown AIDS. Symp-toms may include weight loss of 15% or more of body weight, fever, night sweats, diarrhea, and thrush.

Well-Felix test (Proteus OX-2, OX-K, and OX-19 agglutinins): a test done to determine the presence of typhus and other rickettsial diseases.
Normal values: in serum, four-fold rise in titer between acute and convalescent sera.

Wernicke-Korsakoff syndrome: a group of symp-toms found in people with chronic alcoholism, which include abnormalities of the brain, abnormal eye movements, changes in the pupils of the eye, unstable gait, and psychosis. Treatment consists of vitamins such as thiamine (vitamin B_1), as well as glucose, detoxification, and improved nutrition.

Western blot: a test done on blood to confirm the presence of HIV infection, by finding HIV antibodies in the serum.
Normal value: negative for HIV antibodies

White blood cell count: a count of the white blood cells in a specimen of whole blood.
Normal values: 4500-11,000/mm^3

White blood cell count, differential: a test done on blood to determine the types and proportions of the different types of white blood cells in a specimen of whole blood.
Normal values: (mean; range)
    segmented neutrophils, 56%; 1-7/mL
    bands, 3%; 0-700 μL
    eosinophils, 2.7%; 0-450 μL

basophils, 0.3%; 0-200 μL
lymphocytes, 34%; 1.O-4.8/mL
monocytes, 4%; 0-800 μL

Whooping cough: see Pertussis.

Withdrawal syndrome: a combination of symptoms that develop when a person addicted to a drug or other substance stops taking it.

Wound culture: a culture done on a sample of wound drainage to determine the presence of disease-causing organisms.

— X Y Z —

Xanthochromia: a test done on CSF to determine whether yellow color—due to a breakdown of red blood cells—is present, which may indicate hemorrhage, jaundice, very high protein levels, or a traumatic spinal tap.
Normal value: negative

X-rays (roentgen rays): rays emitted by special equipment that penetrate the body to a calculated depth for diagnostic or treatment purposes.

Xylose absorption test: a test done to determine the rate of absorption of xylose, a wood sugar, into blood. Absorption is impaired in certain disorders of fat absorption.
Normal values:
in serum, 25-40 mg/dL between 1 and 2 hr.
Values in malabsorption:
maximum, approximately 10 mg/dL

Yeast culture: a culture done on cells of vaginal/cervical fluid to detect the presence of yeast infection (candidiasis).
Normal value: no growth of yeast cells

Y chromosome: a gene in sperm, which when present in a fertilized egg determines male sex characteristics and therefore a male child.

Zinc: a metal necessary in trace amounts in body; the level in serum and urine may be elevated in zinc poisoning and some other conditions.
Normal values:
in serum, 70-150 µg/dL;
in urine after 24-hr collection, 0.15-1.2 mg (trace).

Zinc sulfate turbidity test: a test done to determine the gamma globulin concentration in blood; increased in infection, allergy, and autoimmune illnesses, and decreased in some leukemias, cancers, and hypoimmune conditions.
Normal values: in serum, less than 12 U.

Zonography: a technique of tissue layer X-ray study that blurs all tissue layers above and below the layer needed for the study.

Zoonoses: diseases found in animals that are transmissible to humans.

Zygote intrafallopian tube transfer: a method of fertilization in which the fertilized egg (zygote) is placed in the woman's fallopian tube. If all goes well, the egg will travel to the uterus, settle there, and develop into an embryo and fetus.

Measures and Equivalents

Capacity

1 liter (L)	=	1000 milliliters (mL)
1 deciliter (dL)	=	100 milliliters (1/10 L)
1 milliliter (mL)	=	1/1000 liter
1 microliter (µL)	=	1/1,000,000 liter (1/1000 mL)

Weight

1 kilogram (kg)	=	1000 grams (gm)
1 gram (gm)	=	1/1000 kilogram (kg)
1 milligram (mg)	=	1/1000 gram
1 microgram (µg)	=	1/1,000,000 gram
1 nanogram (ng)	=	1/1,000,000,000 gram
1 picogram (pg)	=	1/1,000,000,000,000 gram
1 equivalent (Eq)	=	the weight in grams of the amount of an element that replaces or combines with 1 gram of hydrogen
1 milliequivalent (mEq)	=	1/1000 equivalent
1 microequivalent (µEq)	=	1/1,000,000 equivalent

Length

1 meter (m)	=	39.37 inches (in.)
1 centimeter (cm)	=	1/100 meter
1 millimeter (mm)	=	1/1000 meter
1 micrometer (µm)	=	1/1,000,000 meter
1 nanometer (nm)	=	1/1,000,000,000 meter

Pressure

mm Hg: millimeters of a column of mercury supported by the pressure being measured (used for bodily fluids)

Concentration

milligrams percent (mg%): milligrams per 100 cubic centimeters (cc) or per 100 grams

volume percent (vol%): the number of milliliters of a substance dissolved in 100 milliliters of a liquid

Mols

mol (M): the weight of a substance in grams, equal to its molecular weight; also called gram molecular weight, and mole

millimol (mM): 1/1000 mol

milliosmol (mOsm): unit of osmotic pressure exerted by the concentration of an ion in a solution

molar (M) solution: 1 mol of a substance dissolved in 1 liter of solution

Units

unit (U): an arbitrary measurement used in various laboratory techniques and procedures.

Cherry-Crandall units, mouse uterine units (MUU), Somogyi units, international units, (IU) milli-inter-national units (mIU), Todd units, and the others in this book are unrelated and have different values.

About the Author

Charlotte Isler was Editor of the medical journal *Medical Aspects of Human Sexuality*. She has written many articles on health care, taught writing seminars, and is the author of several books. She is currently writing a book on health, development, and sexuality for teenagers.